Economic evaluation

Understanding Public Health

Series editors: Nick Black and Rosalind Raine, London School of Hygiene & Tropical Medicine

Throughout the world, recognition of the importance of public health to sustainable, safe and healthy societies is growing. The achievements of public health in nineteenth-century Europe were for much of the twentieth century overshadowed by advances in personal care, in particular in hospital care. Now, with the dawning of a new century, there is increasing understanding of the inevitable limits of individual health care and of the need to complement such services with effective public health strategies. Major improvements in people's health will come from controlling communicable diseases, eradicating environmental hazards, improving people's diets and enhancing the availability and quality of effective health care. To achieve this, every country needs a cadre of knowledgeable public health practitioners with social, political and organizational skills to lead and bring about changes at international, national and local levels.

This is one of a series of 20 books that provides a foundation for those wishing to join in and contribute to the twenty-first-century regeneration of public health, helping to put the concerns and perspectives of public health at the heart of policy-making and service provision. While each book stands alone, together they provide a comprehensive account of the three main aims of public health: protecting the public from environmental hazards, improving the health of the public and ensuring high quality health services are available to all. Some of the books focus on methods, others on key topics. They have been written by staff at the London School of Hygiene & Tropical Medicine with considerable experience of teaching public health to students from low, middle and high income countries. Much of the material has been developed and tested with postgraduate students both in face-to-face teaching and through distance learning.

The books are designed for self-directed learning. Each chapter has explicit learning objectives, key terms are highlighted and the text contains many activities to enable the reader to test their own understanding of the ideas and material covered. Written in a clear and accessible style, the series will be essential reading for students taking postgraduate courses in public health and will also be of interest to public health practitioners and policy-makers.

Titles in the series

Analytical models for decision making: Colin Sanderson and Reinhold Gruen
Controlling communicable disease: Norman Noah
Economic analysis for management and policy: Stephen Jan, Lilani Kumaranayake,
 Jenny Roberts, Kara Hanson and Kate Archibald
Economic evaluation: Julia Fox-Rushby and John Cairns (eds)
Environmental epidemiology: Paul Wilkinson (ed)
Environment, health and sustainable development: Megan Landon
Environmental health policy: David Ball (ed)
Financial management in health services: Reinhold Gruen and Anne Howarth
Global change and health: Kelley Lee and Jeff Collin (eds)
Health care evaluation: Sarah Smith, Don Sinclair, Rosalind Raine and Barnaby Reeves
Health promotion practice: Maggie Davies, Wendy Macdowall and Chris Bonell (eds)
Health promotion theory: Maggie Davies and Wendy Macdowall (eds)
Introduction to epidemiology: Lucianne Bailey, Katerina Vardulaki, Julia Langham and
 Daniel Chandramohan
Introduction to health economics: David Wonderling, Reinhold Gruen and Nick Black
Issues in public health: Joceline Pomerleau and Martin McKee (eds)
Making health policy: Kent Buse, Nicholas Mays and Gill Walt
Managing health services: Nick Goodwin, Reinhold Gruen and Valerie Iles
Medical anthropology: Robert Pool and Wenzel Geissler
Principles of social research: Judith Green and John Browne (eds)
Understanding health services: Nick Black and Reinhold Gruen

Economic evaluation

Julia Fox-Rushby and John Cairns (editors)

Open University Press

Open University Press
McGraw-Hill Education
McGraw-Hill House
Shoppenhangers Road
Maidenhead
Berkshire
England
SL6 2QL

email: enquiries@openup.co.uk
world wide web: www.openup.co.uk

and Two Penn Plaza, New York, NY 10121-2289, USA

First published 2005

Copyright © London School of Hygiene & Tropical Medicine

A catalogue record of this book is available from the British Library

ISBN-10: 0 335 21847 4 (pb)
ISBN-13: 978 0 335 21847 9 (pb)

Library of Congress Cataloging-in-Publication Data
CIP data has been applied for

Typeset by RefineCatch Limited, Bungay, Suffolk
Printed and bound by CPI Group (UK) Ltd, Croydon, CR0 4YY

Contents

Acknowledgements

Open University Press and the London School of Hygiene and Tropical Medicine have made every effort to obtain permission from copyright holders to reproduce material in this book and to acknowledge these sources correctly. Any omissions brought to our attention will be remedied in future editions.

We would like to express our grateful thanks to the following copyright holders for granting permission to reproduce material in this book.

p. 98   Acquadro C et al, 'Language and Translation Issues' in Spilker B (ed), *Quality of Life and Pharmacoeconomics in Clinical Trials 2nd edition*. 1996 Lippincott Williams and Wilkins.

p. 80   Attanayake N, Fox-Rushby J and Mills A, 'Household costs of 'malaria' morbidity: a study in Matale district, Sri Lanka,' *Tropical Medicine and International Health*, 5(9): 595–626, Blackwells Publishing Ltd.

p. 24   Reprinted from *Journal of Clinical Epidemiology*, 52(56), Cantor SB and Ganiats TG, 'Incremental cost-effectiveness analysis: the optimal strategy depends in the strategy set,' 517–522, Copyright 1999, with permission from Elsevier.

p. 92   National Centre for Statistics, *Life Tables*. Reproduced by permission of the Centers for Disease Control and prevention.

p. 173   'Modelling the cost effectiveness of lamivudine/zidovudine combination therapy in HIV infection'. *PharmacoEconomics;* 1997, 12(1): 54–66. Figure 1 from page 55. Copyright © 1997 Adis International.

p. 181   Claxton K, 'Bayesian approaches to the value of information: implications for the regulation of new pharmaceuticals,' *Health Economics* 8: 267–274. Copyright 1999. © John Wiley and Sons Limited. Reproduced with permission.

p. 77   Redrawn from Dolan P and Olsen JA (2002), *Distributing Health Care: Economic and Ethical Issues*, by permission of Oxford University Press.

p. 131, 132, 133, 134, 135   Adapted from Donaldson C, Birch S and Gafni A, *The distribution problem in economic evaluation: income and the valuation of costs and consequences of health care programmes*. Copyright 2002. © John Wiley and Sons Limited. Reproduced with permission.

pp. 32–35   Dowie J, '"Evidence-based", "cost-effective" and "preference-driven" medicine: decision analysis based medical decision making is the prerequisite. *J Health Serv Res Policy* 1996; 1: 104–13.

p. 10, 16, 104, 107, 110   Drummond MF, O'Brien B, Stoddart GL and Torrance GW, *Methods for the Economic Evaluation of Health Care Programmes*, 1997. Adapted by permission of Oxford University Press.

pp. 196–203   Dziekan G, et al, 'The cost-effectiveness of policies for the safe and appropriate use of injection healthcare settings,' 2003, *Bulletin of the World Health Organization*, 81(4): 277–285. Adapted by permission of World Health Organization.

p. 95   Fox-Rushby J and Parker M, 'Culture and the measurement of health-related quality of life,' *European Journal of Applied Psychology/Revue Europeene de Psychologie Appliquee*, 45(4): 257–263, Elsevier. Reprinted by permission of Les Editions du Centre de Psychologie Appliquée.

pp. 113, 114–116 Fox-Rushby J, *Disability adjusted life years (DALYs) for decision-making? An overview of the literature*, 2002, Office of Health Economics

pp. 69–70 Nuijten MJC, 'The selection of data sources for use in modelling studies,' in Mallarkey G (ed), *Economic Evaluation in Healthcare*, 1999. Adis International. Copyright Radcliffe Publishing.

pp. 222–24 Rawlins MD, Professor Sir Michael Rawlins' full response to BMJ editorial (2.12.00).

p. 211   Schulman K, Burke J, Drummond M et al, 'Resource costing for multinational neurologic clinical trials: methods and results,' *Health Economics;* 7: 629–638. Copyright 1998. © John Wiley & Sons Limited. Reproduced with permission.

pp. 221–222 Smith R, 'The failings of NICE,' *BMJ*, 2000, 321: 1363–1364, with permission from the BMJ Publishing Group.

p. 146   Reprinted from *Social Science & Medicine*, Vol 37(2), Tormans G, Van Damme P, Carrin G, Clara R, Eylenbusch W, 'Cost-effectiveness analysis of perinatal screening and vaccination against hepatitis B virus – the case of Belgium', 173–181, copyright 1993, with permission from Elsevier.

p. 138   Reprinted from *Social Science and Medicine*, Vol 48(2), Tsuchiya A, 'Age-related preferences and age weighting health benefits', 267–276, copyright 1999, with permission from Elsevier.

pp. 163–67, 169 Walker D and Fox-Rushby J, 'Allowing for uncertainty in economic evaluations: qualitative sensitivity analysis,' *Health Policy and Planning*, 2001, 16(4): 435–443, by permission of Oxford University Press.

pp. 26–27 Walker D, McDermott JM, Fox-Rushby J et al, 'An economic analysis of midwifery training programmes in South Kalimantan, Indonesia,' *Bulletin of the World Health Organization*, 80(1): 47–55. Reprinted with permission of World Health Organization.

Overview of the book

Introduction

There are so many ways in which health might be improved today and, as technology improves, the opportunities will increase. However, governments, health care providers and families can't have or do everything because they face a number of constraints. There are limits to budgets as well as other resources (such as the number of specialists or laboratories available). Therefore, choices have to be made about what to spend money and time on. Economic evaluation can help set out what the value of costs and benefits from competing choices are.

This book gives you an introductory working knowledge of economic evaluation. It provides a range of tools as well as a structure for thinking about how to evaluate and improve the value for money from spending on health care. Whilst the use of techniques for costing, valuing benefits and analysing data are introduced, you are encouraged to take a critical view of such activities. What you will realize by the end of the book is that any economic evaluation is as much a matter of art as it is of science and, like any artist, what an evaluator perceives will influence the final picture. In practice the skills of an economist and the quality of an economic evaluation will depend on collaboration with health care professionals, epidemiologists, statisticians and other social scientists. You are therefore encouraged to develop the talents of a critic, draw on your wider knowledge and unlock the key to developing useful economic evaluations – working out who wants to use the information for what decision.

Why study economic evaluation?

Other than giving value to the pursuit of knowledge, you may have a variety of reasons such as:

- the increasing role of economic evaluation in influencing funding decisions and guidance in international health policy such as by the World Health Organization (WHO);
- the increasing likelihood that considerations of cost-effectiveness will be incorporated within clinical guidelines;
- the possibility of economic evaluation being introduced as the 'fourth hurdle' in the evaluation of medicines and devices following three regulatory procedures (quality, safety and efficacy; review and approval of registration for human use; negotiations about pricing and reimbursement);
- the use of cost-effectiveness as a marketing tool by the pharmaceutical industry;
- the need to interpret treatment guidelines based on cost-effectiveness at national and sub-national levels;

- wanting to commission and be a critical consumer of the results of economic evaluations;
- to find out how (and whose) values and judgements enter into economic analyses;
- to plan an economic evaluation in practice; or
- to help make decisions more accountable.

Structure of the book

This book is similar to the 'economic evaluation' teaching unit at the London School of Hygiene & Tropical Medicine. It is partly based on the materials presented in the lectures and seminars of that course.

The book is in five sections. It begins by setting out ways in which economic evaluations might be structured and moves on to consider approaches to measuring and valuing costs, and then the outcomes of health care interventions. The fourth section is the presentation and interpretation of evidence. The final section critically appraises the usefulness of economic evaluation in practice, policy, and as a method and way of thinking.

The five sections, and the 20 chapters within them, are shown on the book's contents page. Each chapter, as appropriate, includes:

- an overview;
- a list of learning objectives;
- a list of key terms;
- a range of activities;
- feedback on the activities;
- a summary;
- references and further reading.

Although examples and case studies in this book are balanced between interests of low-, middle- and high-income countries, you should be aware that most of the theory on economic evaluation has been derived in high-income countries.

The following description of the contents of each section and chapter will give you an idea of what you will be studying.

The structure of economic evaluation

The framework of any study of efficiency affects the research questions posed, data gathered and interpretations that can be given to the evidence. Therefore, the first chapter sets out how different types of economic evaluation can address alternative concepts of efficiency, followed in Chapter 2 with a set of key issues that determine the structure of economic evaluations. Decision analysis is a useful framework on which to structure and build economic evaluations and this is introduced in Chapter 3. Chapters 4 and 5 then work through the two most common approaches to decision analysis: decision-trees and Markov models.

Measuring and valuing resource use

A fundamental part of any economic evaluation is estimating the quantity and value of resource use between competing alternatives. This includes both the value of resources used to implement an intervention as well as the value of resources that can be saved and used for something else. Chapter 6 describes and discusses issues in measuring and valuing resources within health services and Chapter 7 considers non-health service costs (e.g. the impact on patients or families and productivity). Both chapters consider the range of primary and secondary sources of data.

Measuring and valuing consequences

Chapter 8 gets you to think about all the possible consequences of health care interventions and how to decide what to measure in an economic evaluation. Having measured the physical quantities of health change, Chapter 9 introduces you to different ways of valuing changes in health without using money and asks you to consider the uses and challenges. Chapter 10 asks you to consider how to account for the combination of health and non-health effects that could arise from health care interventions and what monetary values can and can't reflect. Chapter 11 reviews the equity implications of approaches to valuation and considers how it might be measured and accounted for. The final chapter describes the principles and practice of discounting both benefits and cost consequences.

Presenting and interpreting the evidence

Chapter 13 considers the summary measures used to report cost-effectiveness analyses and how they can be used to inform decision-making. Together with a basic sensitivity analysis presented in Chapter 14, this would represent the minimum requirements expected in presenting the results of any economic evaluation. Chapter 15 develops the role of sensitivity analysis for an individual analysis to include probabilistic sensitivity analysis and how this might help interpretations if developed to include cost-effectiveness planes and net benefit analyses. Chapter 16 outlines the different ways in which data are most commonly presented and requested.

Appraising the quality and usefulness of economic evaluation

It is important for any study to produce valid results for the context and purpose of the evaluation, although in practice the results of evaluations are not always used in one setting. Therefore, Chapter 17 helps you develop a critique of a specific study and Chapter 18 works through alternative approaches to transferring results across settings. Chapter 19 takes a critical look at the quality of economic evaluations in practice and their use to decision-makers at the local, national or international level. The final chapter takes a critical look at economic evaluation as a whole, drawing on criticisms within and outside economics.

It is always good to read around a subject and keep up to date with current developments. The most consistently useful journal publishing on the theory, methodology and application of economic evaluation is *Health Economics*. Other journals that publish regularly on theory and methodology include the *Journal of Health Economics, Medical Decision Making, Medical Care* and *Social Science and Medicine*. In addition, applications of economic evaluation appear in the *Journal of Health Services Research & Policy, Health Policy, European Journal of Health Economics, International Journal of Technology Assessment in Health Care, Applied Health Economics and Health Policy, Health Policy and Planning, Cost-Effectiveness and Resource Allocation* and *Pharmacoeconomics*.

The internet is also a useful source for further information. You may find the following of particular use in supplementing your knowledge on economic evaluation: a searchable database reviewing over 2000 economic evaluations, with the following web address: http://www.york.ac.uk/inst/crd/nhsdhp.htm; and a series of downloadable reports evaluating the effectiveness and efficiency of specific health interventions in the UK. A CD with all these reports is available free worldwide: http://www.ncchta.org/ProjectData/3_publication_listings_ALL.asp

Authors

Julia Fox-Rushby is Professor of Health Economics, Boyka Stoykova is a Research Fellow and Alec Miners is an Honorary Research Fellow at Brunel University; John Cairns is Professor of Health Economics, Damian Walker is a Lecturer in Health Economics, Jo-Ann Mulligan is a Research Fellow, and Dogan Fidan is an Honorary Research Fellow at the London School of Hygiene & Tropical Medicine.

Acknowledgements

We thank Catriona Waddington for reviewing the final manuscript and Deirdre Byrne, series manager, for help and support.

SECTION 1

The structure of economic evaluation

Efficiency and economic evaluation

Overview

In this chapter you will learn about how different economic evaluations can help address policy questions that seek to improve the efficiency of investments in health care. You will learn that different types of efficiency and economic evaluation exist and see why economic evaluations may provide different results as a consequence of comparing different interventions, the viewpoint of analysis and construction of total costs and consequences. You will also be introduced to the links in the pursuit of equity.

Learning objectives

After working through this chapter, you will be able to:

- **describe how economic evaluation can contribute to different types of policy questions**
- **distinguish different forms of economic evaluation**
- **explain how economic evaluation is related to assessing efficiency**
- **understand the comparative basis of economic evaluation**
- **distinguish alternative numerators and denominators for use in economic evaluation**

Key terms

Allocative (Pareto, social) efficiency A situation in which it is not possible to improve the welfare of one person in an economy without making someone else worse off.

Average cost-effectiveness ratio The total cost divided by total effectiveness of a single intervention (where effectiveness is measured on a single scale).

Comparator An alternative against which a new intervention is compared.

Disability adjusted life year (DALY) A measure to adjust life years lived for disease related disability, age and time preference.

Equity Fairness, defined in terms of equality of opportunity, provision, use or outcome.

Incremental cost-effectiveness ratio (ICER) The ratio of the difference in cost between two alternatives to the difference in effectiveness between the same two alternatives.

Marginal cost The change in the total cost if one additional unit of output is produced.

Marginal social benefit The extra benefit from consumption of a good as viewed by society as a whole.

Marginal social cost The cost that the production of another unit of output imposes on society.

Operational (technical, productive) efficiency Using only the minimum necessary resources to finance, purchase and deliver a particular activity or set of activities (ie avoiding waste).

Opportunity (economic) cost The value of the next best alternative foregone as a result of the decision made.

Quality Adjusted Life Years (QALYs) A year of life adjusted for its quality or its value. A year in perfect health is considered equal to 1.0 QALY.

Systematic review A review of the literature that uses an explicit approach to searching, selecting and combining the relevant studies.

What is economic evaluation and how important is it?

Economic evaluations compare the costs and consequences of two (or more) health care interventions. Economic evaluation is a way of thinking, backed up by a set of tools, which is designed to improve the value for money from investments in health care and welfare.

The reason economic evaluation is needed is because markets alone do not provide efficient solutions, particularly in health care. However, when free markets don't exist, active decisions have to be made about which health services should be funded given the scarce resources available. This scarcity includes time, technology, capital and labour inputs as well as monetary budgets. The overall aim is to maximize benefits given the resources available.

After a brief look at any newspaper you are likely to find that government decision-makers and large private sector companies are claiming, or seeking, increases in efficiency, for example by increasing output, increasing the welfare of the population or cutting costs. Decision-makers often have to make very difficult decisions, especially when technology is constantly improving. Below you will find examples of a number of statements made about the need to provide malaria vaccines and other services that offer value for money. It is so important that, even though it is likely that malaria vaccines are not going to be available for ten years, national and international agencies are already beginning to consider the issue:

The [WHO] strategy recognises that malaria varies throughout the world, with the consequences that cost-effectiveness control must be based on local analysis.

(WHO 2005)

World Bank president James Wolfensohn recently told the *Financial Times* that the Bank plans to create a $1 billion fund to help countries purchase specified vaccines if and when they are developed . . . The program would be highly focused on areas of deep poverty and would be highly cost effective.

(Glennerster and Kremer 2000)

Strategic decisions, under the significant resource constraints that exist in developing countries, should be determined not only by the burden of disease among the poor but also the cost-effectiveness of health interventions in terms of the health benefits gained.

(DfID 2000)

Improving public expenditure management . . . requires that government expenditures pass the litmus test of cost-effectiveness to ensure value for money and reduce extravagance.

(Ghana Poverty Reduction Strategy 2002)

Health policy and investment decisions are taken by a wide variety of different agencies. At a national level, policy-makers within ministries of health and finance will be concerned with allocating budgets across various competing needs (e.g. health versus education, reducing malaria versus diarrhoeal diseases, providing preventive vaccines versus treatment of disease). At the global level, agencies might provide:

- direct funding of interventions (e.g. Global Alliance for Vaccines Initiative and the Vaccine Fund, World Bank health sector and development loans, bi-lateral aid);
- guidance and funding for research (e.g. the Malaria Vaccine Initiative's role in accelerating the development of promising malaria vaccines);
- guidance for policy (e.g. the WHO's role in setting recommended vaccination schedules and influencing strategic policies of 'Roll Back Malaria').

Each type of decision will require different information but there are some key ideas that each will be interested in: what will be the costs and consequences of changes to current practice? How reliable are the predictions of changes in costs and benefits? And is the change 'worth it'? Differences in budgets, health care practices and epidemiological and economic environments can affect whether policies should change at a specific point in time and in a specific country.

Types of economic evaluation

Table 1.1 shows that there are different types of evaluation which can be used to answer different decision questions. Whilst each approach measures costs in terms of money, they differ in the way that consequences are included. Cost-benefit analysis (CBA) is the only type of economic evaluation to put costs and benefits in monetary terms and it is therefore able to compare interventions across sectors as well as help decide how much money to invest in a programme. Using CBA implies placing a value on life and health, which is difficult (see Chapter 12). Partly because of the difficulties of valuing benefits and partly because decision-makers can find a single amount representing costs and benefits from a programme disconcertingly impenetrable, cost-consequence analysis (CCA) was developed. CCA ensures that health and non-health outcomes are identified and quantified

Table 1.1 Differentiating types of economic evaluation

Types of economic evaluation	Cost measure	Type of consequences identified for all alternatives	Methods for measuring and valuing consequences	Type of efficiency	Decision context: malaria vaccine relative to ...
Cost-minimization analysis	Money	Clinical or health effect needs to be identical between options	None	Technical	Alternative malaria vaccines or other malaria prevention strategies
Cost-consequence analysis	Money	Clinical, health and non-health impacts	Listing of separate consequences with no comparable valuation	Technical	Other (non-health) public sector investments (but no decision rule)
Cost-effectiveness analysis	Money	One single clinical or health effect of interest to both alternatives	Number fully vaccinated children, cases averted, life years gained	Technical	Alternative malaria vaccines or other malaria control interventions
Cost-utility analysis	Money	Single or multiple effects, not necessarily common to both alternatives	DALYs averted or QALYs gained	Technical, moving to allocative within the health sector only	Other health sector interventions
Cost-benefit analysis	Money	Single or multiple effects, not necessarily common to both alternatives	Money	Allocative	Other (non-health) public sector investments

Source: Adapted from Drummond et al 1997

even though they are not valued. However, these two approaches offer decision-makers very different help: CBA is the only method that can be used to argue for more resources to the health sector and CCA is the only method without a clear decision rule.

Cost-effectiveness analysis (CEA) (and cost-minimization analysis, CMA, as a specific subset of cost-effectiveness analysis) is the most frequently used form of economic evaluation in the health sector. It can be applied to many different types of health programme as the outcome measures used can easily vary. However, one of the limitations is that CEA only focuses on a single outcome common to the alternatives being evaluated. Therefore, it can't be used to compare across programmes that affect different outcomes without missing many of the effects, and a common outcome may not be considered the primary outcome of interest to both alternatives.

Quality adjusted life years (QALYs) and disability adjusted life years (DALYs) are different ways of adjusting life expectancy for the quality of life lived during those years. These measures significantly increase the usefulness of economic evaluation because different interventions can be compared and multiple effects on quality of life can also be included. This has led to the development of a form of economic evaluation specific to the health sector: cost-utility analysis (CUA). CUA can compare a broader range of health care programmes than CEA. Ultimately, QALYs are a more flexible measure as they can capture the impact of any disease, whereas DALYs are calculated separately for single diseases and don't allow consideration of additional diseases. This and other issues are covered in more detail in Chapter 9.

 Activity 1.1

Listed below are a series of policy questions. Which type of economic evaluation do you think would be best to use and why?

1 The Ministry of Health wants to know whether to invest in fixed-site or mobile clinics for cataract surgery.
2 The Ministry of Finance wants to know how much money to allocate to immunization over the next five years.
3 The Ministry of Health wants to know whether they should switch to providing a new drug as the first line treatment for malaria.
4 The district health officer wants to know whether the district should adopt the WHO recommended guidelines for the content and number of antenatal care visits, given that there was no significant difference in outcomes for the WHO package of care compared with current practice in Argentina, Saudi Arabia, Thailand or Cuba (assuming an average of five antenatal appointments per pregnancy) (Villar et al. 2001).
5 Should a hospital manager introduce a new but expensive drug that does not improve health but does reduce the length of hospital stay?

Feedback

1 CMA if outcomes are the same but CEA if not – or CUA if sufficient data are available on change in morbidity and mortality.

2 CBA because of deciding on the size of the budget.

3 CUA as there are differences in morbidity and mortality.

4 CMA can be used as there was no difference in outcomes. However, if the average number of antenatal care visits in a country is less than five, a CEA would be needed as this would increase the number of visits required.

5 CMA provided there is no worsening of health.

Table 1.1 also indicates that the nature of efficiency differs by type of economic evaluation. CCA, CMA and CEA address technical efficiency. Achieving technical efficiency requires that outputs are maximized from the resources available and also produced at minimum cost. Figure 1.1 demonstrates positions of efficiency and inefficiency. You can work through it in two stages.

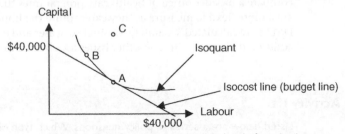

Points A, B, & C represent the same level of production.

Figure 1.1 Points of technical (in)efficiency

First, look at the isoquant line ('iso' meaning 'the same' and 'quant' meaning the 'quantity' of output) which indicates the minimum number of resources needed to produce one level of output, say a surgical operation. Points A and B produce the same output but require different mixes of labour and capital. Point C, which, in this case, also produces the same output, is not efficient because it takes more capital and more labour than B to produce the same surgical operation.

Second, look at the isocost line – also known as the 'budget line'. Costs are equal all along this line. If you knew a budget was $40,000, then you could draw a budget line. For example, if the $40,000 were all spent on capital this would equal the point on the vertical axis and if the $40,000 were all spent on labour this would equal the point on the horizontal axis. The budget line is then drawn between these two points and, as you go down the line, more labour is bought and less capital, but the cost remains the same. The point at which the isoquant and isocost touch is the point of technical efficiency – the point where the maximum is produced at minimum cost. You can see this by working out what point B means; whilst B represents an efficient mix of inputs, it lies beyond the budget line and is therefore not affordable.

✎ **Activity 1.2**

Figure 1.2 shows the level of efficiency achieved by alternative ways of treating acute angina (chest pain). Explain why long hospitalization in a general hospital is more efficient than a teaching hospital but not when compared with a shorter stay.

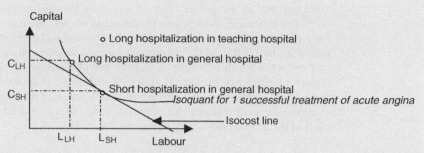

Figure 1.2 Comparison of hospitalization type

Source: LSHTM

Feedback

Long hospitalization in a general hospital is technically efficient as it lies on the isoquant (unlike the teaching hospital which requires more capital and more labour to produce the same output). However, as the point lies to the right of the budget line it indicates that long hospitalization costs more than short hospitalization and therefore is not an economically efficient option. In this example, note that you are assuming that output is identical. For example, if quality of life were higher amongst patients who had long hospitalization, this answer would not hold. Note also that any costs falling on patients are ignored as this analysis is conducted from the perspective of a hospital only.

Allocative efficiency moves beyond considering the best way to achieve a set goal within a given budget to judging whether the goal itself is worthwhile. CBA addresses allocative efficiency. Once the production side of health care is technically efficient, this form of efficiency considers efficiency from the wider viewpoint of society. It therefore assesses whether:

- changing the mix of suppliers could increase production;
- changing the mix of consumers could increase overall satisfaction (referred to by economists as *utility*).

Allocative efficiency is achieved when no resources are wasted and when it is not possible to make one person better off without making another worse off. A market is efficient if it is producing the right goods for the right people at the right price. In health care, because prices may not exist, this translates to ensuring that, for the last unit consumed, marginal social benefit is exactly equal to marginal social cost.

Table 1.1 began to indicate that linking the types of economic evaluation and efficiency was not entirely straightforward and the main difficulty is with CUA. QALYs and DALYs both seek to encapsulate patients' values. For example, QALYs are based on studies that ask individuals about their preferences for different combinations of outcomes. This clearly goes beyond efficient production and moves you towards allocative efficiency. However, because QALYs and DALYs only consider health and disease, they don't allow comparison across sectors (e.g. housing, transport) and therefore can't be used to assess efficiency from the point of view of the whole economy. A second, less obvious, challenge concerns not the theory of efficiency but the practice of economic evaluation. Whilst CEA, for example, theoretically considers technical efficiency, in practice few studies seek to examine the most efficient way of maximizing outputs and minimizing costs from each of the interventions they compare.

Economic evaluation as comparison

The opening statement of this chapter highlighted the comparative nature of economic evaluation. Comparison occurs between (at least) two interventions and between costs and consequences. Table 1.1 will have given you some idea that the comparators for an economic evaluation can differ substantially and the interventions compared will partly depend on the questions being asked by decision-makers. However, comparisons selected can themselves limit the decisions made.

There are two ways in which interventions can be compared:

- Within a single analysis, as most frequently occurs in CEA. An example would include a comparison of the costs and consequences of vaccinating children for malaria versus giving no vaccination in terms of preventing severe malaria.
- Within a single analysis and by comparing results across findings from several studies, as most frequently occurs with CUA. An example would include using the example from above but evaluating the consequences of a malaria vaccine in terms of DALYs averted or QALYs gained. Once the analysis is completed, the results would be comparable with findings from other interventions designed to improve health, such as improving water and sanitation, even though the alternatives were not considered in the original study. The broader the outcome measure used, the more widely interventions can be compared.

This idea of comparison is fundamental and is related to the way in which economists estimate the value or worth of something. Economic evaluation is a formal way of valuing an intervention in terms of opportunity cost. Opportunity cost is a way of valuing a good or service in terms of what had to be sacrificed in order to obtain that item – that is why comparison amongst options and of costs and consequences is so important. It is also the basis for valuing individual costs and consequences within any intervention.

✎ Activity 1.3

Imagine that intervention A is the introduction of a childhood vaccination programme for hepatitis B (a viral infection of the liver). What alternative interventions might you want to compare this against?

○✓ **Feedback**

The costs and consequences could be compared against one of more of the following:

*   doing nothing (i.e. not giving hepatitis B vaccination)
*   vaccinating only health workers for hepatitis B
*   treating hepatitis B
*   introducing a hib vaccine (which protects against infection)
*   extending coverage of existing vaccines

These examples consider some options within the vaccination field and you may have thought of others. However, comparisons could also go beyond vaccination to consider other child or adult health programmes (e.g. impregnated mosquito nets or mobile mammography clinics) and also go beyond the health sector (e.g. primary education). The choice of options will depend on the needs of the decision-maker.

Economic evaluation also compares the costs and consequences of interventions. Figure 1.3 shows that two types of ratio can be calculated from any economic evaluation: average cost-effectiveness ratios (ACERs) and incremental cost-effectiveness ratios (ICERs). ACERs relate to single interventions. The marginal cost (the extra cost of producing one extra output or outcome) can be estimated from these ratios. However, because economic evaluation is a comparative analysis, results should focus on presenting ICERs – that is, the difference in costs incurred by moving from one intervention to another divided by the difference in consequences from moving from one intervention to another. The ICER is therefore a relative measure, and the choice of comparator for a new intervention is clearly influential. You will learn in Chapter 2 how to choose appropriate comparators.

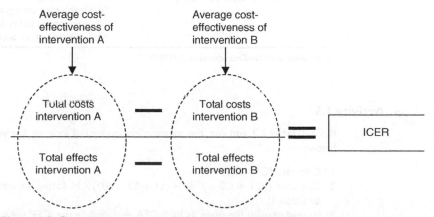

Figure 1.3 Components in a comparative economic evaluation

Activity 1.4

Here is a brief summary of results by Scott *et al.* (2004) on the economic cost of pneumonia acquired in the community (rather than in hospital) among adults in New Zealand. Why is it not an economic evaluation and what additional information would be needed to turn it into an economic evaluation?

'It was estimated that in 2003 there were 26,826 episodes of pneumonia in adults; a rate of 859 per 100,000 people. The annual cost was estimated to be 63 million dollars (direct medical costs of 29 million dollars; direct non-medical costs of 1 million dollars; lost productivity of 33 million dollars).'

 Feedback

This is a cost of illness study, not an economic evaluation, because the costs of care are not compared between two methods for preventing, caring for or treating people with pneumonia.

Whilst a comparison of costs and consequences appears relatively straightforward, there is one note of caution. Both the numerator and denominator might include different components. Therefore, when comparing studies, it is also important to check what costs and consequences are included and how. Table 1.2 outlines components of costs and consequences that could be incorporated in an economic evaluation depending on the viewpoint. An evaluation adopting a societal view-point would need to include C1, C2 and C3 costs whereas an evaluation from the perspective of the health service need only include C1.

Table 1.2 Costs and consequences

Net costs	Net consequences
C1 Health care costs (£50 000)	Health (H): 400 years of life gained
C2 Patient & family costs (£3000)	Utility (U): 290 QALYs
C3 Cost in other sectors (£10 000)	WTPU: Willingness to pay (£2000 000)
	S1: Health care savings (£5000)
	S2: Savings to patients & families (£2000)
	S3: Savings to other sectors (£4000)

Source: Adapted from Drummond *et al.* (1997)

 Activity 1.5

Review Table 1.2 and use the information presented in it to answer the questions below.

1 Calculate (C1 − S1) / H.
2 Calculate ((C1 + C2 + C3) − (S1 + S2 + S3)) / H (compare with the answer to question 1).
3 Instead of using life years, as for a CEA, re-calculate the ICER for a CUA.

4 Give two alternative formulae for calculating values of net benefit for CBA.
5 Reflect on your results and consider what impact the differences in viewpoint and
   choice of outcome measure is likely to have.
6 In what circumstance might a negative cost-effectiveness ratio exist (i.e. a net saving
   in costs and health benefits)?

↻ Feedback

1 (£50,000 − £5000) / 400 life years gained = £112.5 per life year gained.

2 ((£50,000 + 3000 + 10,000) − (£5000 + 2000 + 4000)) / 400 life years gained = £130
per life year gained.

3 (£50,000 − £5000) / 290 QALYs gained = £155.2 per QALY gained.

4 WTPU − (C1 + C2 + C3) or, alternatively, (WTPU + S1 + S2 + S3) − (C1 + C2 + C3).

5 The differences could make it difficult to compare results across studies and affect
the decision to adopt an intervention.

6 A negative ICER would exist if the costs saved from reductions in treatment costs
exceeded the costs of putting an intervention in place and if that intervention also
conferred additional health benefits. Examples in the past have included introducing
immunization programmes in some countries.

How are economic evaluations designed and conducted?

There are two broad approaches to undertaking economic evaluations: those that
collect new (primary) data as part of randomized clinical trials or non-randomized
studies (such as before and after studies or comparison of two geographic areas);
and those that rely on existing (secondary) data, or existing studies. Both may also
involve modelling. For example, randomized trials may not last long enough to
capture all the consequences of an intervention so these need to be modelled.
Alternatively, a model may produce results that are so uncertain that particular
data need to be collected. You will be learning about the nature and sources of data
available for both costs and consequences and reviewing both the role and practice
of modelling and randomized trials in later chapters.

A final note on equity

Economic evaluation is first and foremost an analysis of equity. There are two ways
in which equity might be accounted for. First, the principles of cost-effectiveness
can be used to assess which is the most efficient route to achieving equity.
Second, weights might be used to revalue data on consequences, such that greater
weight is given to certain members of a population. All techniques covered in this
book are relevant to equipping you with relevant knowledge for the first option.
With respect to the second option, you are likely to find Chapters 11 and 20 most
useful.

Summary

Economic evaluation assesses the value for money from investing in health care interventions. This analysis of efficiency compares the costs and consequences of interventions. The interventions compared can be very closely related to each other or not, depending on the way in which consequences are accounted for. The more widely the consequences of interventions are considered, the more helpful to decision-makers who have to allocate budgets to, and within, the health sector. As economic evaluations are indicators of relative efficiency and because ICERs can be constructed with different information, it is important to be able to understand their meaning before making policy recommendations.

References

DfID (2000) *Better health for poor people*. London: Department for International Development.

Drummond MF, O'Brien B, Stoddart GL and Torrance GW (1997) *Methods for the economic evaluation of health care programmes*. Oxford: Oxford Medical Publications, Chapter 2.

Ghana Poverty Reduction Strategy (2002) final draft version, 20 February, www.dfid.gov.uk/pubs/files/ghana-pov-red-strat.pdf.

Glennerster G and Kremer M (2000) *A World Bank vaccine commitment*, policy briefing no. 57, Brookings Institute, www.brookings.org/comm/policybriefs/pb57.htm.

Scott G, Scott H, Turley M and Baker M (2004) Economic cost of community-acquired pneumonia in New Zealand adults. *NZ Med J*. 117(1196).

WHO (2005) *Current recommendations: malaria control today*. Geneva: WHO.

Further reading

Dinwiddy C and Teal F (1996) *Principles of cost-benefit analysis for developing countries*. Cambridge: Cambridge University Press, Chapters 1–3.

2 | Framing an economic evaluation

Overview

In this chapter you will be introduced to the range of possibilities for framing economic evaluations and consider the implications of each frame for the estimated cost-effectiveness ratios.

Learning objectives

After working through this chapter, you will be able to:

- list at least six issues to consider in framing an economic evaluation
- offer different ways each issue could be used to frame an economic evaluation
- understand the importance of being able to describe who does what, to whom, where and how often for all options considered
- form a full question for an economic evaluation
- discuss the potential implications of different frames of reference on the cost-effectiveness ratios and the policy decisions, and effects of the decisions on health providers, funders and patients/families

Key terms

Clinical guidelines Advice based on the best available research evidence and clinical expertise.

Gold standard A method, procedure or measurement that is widely accepted as being the best available (nearest the truth).

Managed care organization Health care provider that offers comprehensive health services based on explicit clinical guidelines.

Introduction

At the beginning of an economic evaluation, you need to set and justify the boundaries for the study. This includes specifying the research question, the analytical approach, the options for comparison, and the approach to costs and outcomes.

Early consideration of these issues is important as decisions affect which data are collected, how they are analysed and how policy options are interpreted. Making inappropriate choices with respect to viewpoint or comparators, missing costs or focusing on the wrong time period could lead to inefficient decisions if results are implemented or, at best, result in wasted research.

Choices should be guided by how information will be used. Careful consideration of the issues and careful documenting of the assumptions made at the beginning of an evaluation can also help guide sensitivity analysis as well as a discussion of the contribution and limitations of a study.

Hill *et al.* (2000) reviewed all major submissions to the Department of Health and Aged Care in Australia and found that, of the 326 submissions, 67% had significant problems, over half of which were considered 'avoidable' – which included 15 for which there was disagreement over the choice of the comparator. Walker and Fox-Rushby (2000) raised similar concerns in their review of economic evaluations of communicable disease interventions in low-income countries. They found that only 25/107 stated the perspective of the analysis and that whilst authors describe a new option they fail to describe adequately the comparator (which is often existing practice). This reduces the extent to which results can be interpreted reliably across countries or over time, as practices vary.

The key points you will consider in setting the framework for an economic evaluation are:

- objectives of the analysis;
- audience for the evaluation;
- viewpoint of the analysis;
- analytic horizon;
- specify the intervention;
- specify the alternative intervention(s) for comparison;
- target population.

Objectives of the analysis

To use scarce research resources effectively, you need to understand the decision context of a study. For example, is an evaluation just intended to contribute to the evidence in an area or are the results needed to make a specific decision? This requires thinking about who the audience for the evaluation is, who contributes to the policy process, and their issues of interest (such as current practices and the information stakeholders are likely to draw).

Torrance *et al.* (1996) distinguish 'what is' and 'what if' studies, with the former tending to have more and better quality data and the latter addressing issues before good data are available but when a policy decision is still needed. There may be particularly important individual studies, a meta-analysis or evaluations from specific countries that are considered more important in 'what is' evaluations. Alternatively, because 'what if' studies offer good opportunities to use threshold analyses for examining how the size of costs and effects might affect a decision (see Chapter 14), you should find out which variables decision-makers are most concerned about (and judge which ones they have some control over).

It is important to think ahead about what the results of an evaluation will be compared against. This should not only affect the choice of comparators within a study but might also affect which costs and outcomes are selected. For example, if decision-makers consider a particular study as the 'gold standard', then it may be important to measure the same inputs and outcomes, or use the same population group, or use the same reference costs to value resources. Alternatively, if a judgement on what constitutes an important clinical difference (the smallest change in health status that patients perceive as significant and which could justify a change in a patient's management) has been made, then you should include such a measure in your study.

Audience for the evaluation

The main audience for an evaluation should be the principal users – the people making a decision with the information, who may be different from the funders of the evaluation. This can include:

- government (e.g. Ministry of Health or specific hospitals);
- managed care organizations (e.g. Kaiser Permanente in California);
- international organizations (e.g. World Bank, WHO);
- bilateral aid agencies (e.g. JICA, SIDA);
- non-governmental aid agencies (e.g. Action Aid, Medecin Sans Frontiers);
- pharmaceutical companies.

These organizations may have different requirements. For example, the National Institute for Health and Clinical Excellence (NICE) in the UK and the Canadian Coordinating Office for Health Technology Assessment have different guidelines for evaluations (see Chapter 13). Sometimes evaluations will just add to general knowledge rather than being targeted to specific decision-makers or alternatively, have results of interest to secondary groups. For example, evaluating a malaria control scheme that involves draining land will be of interest to the Ministries of Health and Agriculture as well as local councils and the community. Identifying the audience helps decide which methods are best used, as well as the best reporting format.

Viewpoint (or perspective) of the analysis

The perspective of the analysis is the viewpoint you use to examine the question and this affects which types of costs and outcomes are included and how they are valued. The two types of perspective to choose from are:

- society; or,
- decision-makers, e.g. government (national, regional or local), health care providers, third-party payers, businesses, patients and families.

The societal perspective is the broadest and considers all costs and benefits regardless of who pays for or receives them. It is limited by selecting a specific geographical area but usually focuses on whole countries. Gold *et al.* (1996) recommend that studies that aim to address the appropriate allocation of resources should adopt a societal perspective because all costs are considered even if different interventions shift them from one group (e.g. hospitals) to another (e.g. family doctors). One important implication is that opportunity costs are the appropriate method for valuing resources (see Chapter 1) and the general public for valuing benefits (see Chapters 8 and 9).

Decision-makers often belong to a specific organization and may therefore wish to conduct an evaluation from a narrower perspective. For example:

* the manager of a coronary heart disease programme may be more interested in who is paying for new equipment than the societal cost;
* a business may want to know about the impact on its own workforce of providing treatment and prevention for HIV;
* the manager of a mosquito bednet distribution programme may not be interested in the impact the programme has on a community health worker's other activities.

Adopting one perspective does not preclude another and you can choose to adopt a narrower and societal perspective, and present two sets of results. However, it is important to recognize the different political incentives at stake and that public sector decision-makers at the central level will have to review the results of evaluations carefully to ensure that their objectives are met. This might, for example, include a requirement that the costs borne by patients in accessing new health services are fully accounted for to ensure that costs are not shifted and 'hidden', or to be aware of the opportunity cost of pursuing policies that seek equity.

Analytic horizon

The analytic horizon is the period of time covered by the analysis. It should be selected to:

* cover all the main costs and benefits that are incurred;
* allow for any seasonal or other cyclical variation;
* cover the period over which an intervention is set up, implemented and run.

Costs and benefits may occur at different periods of time (e.g. costs of improving the quality of blood supplies may be incurred immediately but the benefits reaped over a lifetime, especially as some lives will be saved). The analytical horizon needs to be long enough to cover both. This often means having to model costs and outcomes beyond the period for which primary data are available.

Specifying the intervention(s)

The interventions to be analysed and the system within which it is delivered need to be described fully and with care. This will help ensure that all resources used are identified and allow others to understand exactly what was evaluated, which is important for considering the generalizability of the results.

The more complex the intervention, the more complex the description will be. However, it is important to stress that evidence on effectiveness will be needed for each intervention evaluated and thus some interventions may have to be excluded. Reviewing many options greatly complicates analysis.

Drummond *et al.* (1997) provide a helpful list of issues to describe interventions.

They suggest that to identify costs you need to ask who does what, to whom, where and how often and to identify consequences you need to ask what are the results? In responding to these questions evaluators should consider relevant activities in providing care as well as in setting up, monitoring and managing the new interventions.

Who?

Personnel are often a high proportion of costs and use of labour can differ between countries. Therefore, the types of people providing care should be described. For example, care may be provided by doctors, nurses or members of the community and management by programme managers. All the contributors to the intervention should be described (both funders and providers) as this can help identify types of costs and sources of data needed for the evaluation.

Does what?

Describe all the different activities associated with each intervention. This might include a clinical protocol as well as any new training required in setting up an intervention or supervisory visits.

To whom?

The ages and types of patients (including co-morbidities and risk factors) should be described. If interventions are divided into different groups (e.g. by age or risk factor), then each should be described.

Where?

Explain where each part of the intervention is delivered – for example, within a health centre or the type of hospital. If an intervention covers care in many settings, this should be described as well as the typical pathways of care. A description should also include whether the intervention evaluated is delivered on its own or alongside other services (health, social care etc.). A description of the management structure may need to outline the different levels of health system involved (e.g. if district or regional health managers have a role).

How often?

This should cover the:

- period of time over which the intervention is expected to operate – for example, evaluations might consider a one-year period or running a service for a group of patients from birth to death;
- frequency with which individuals or specific groups of patients are seen – for example, an intervention may categorize treatment paths by risk group.

What are the results?

First, good practice requires that all consequences of an intervention are identified. The second task is to decide which consequences are measurable and how, and following this, how the consequences measured should be valued. This not only helps clarify how comprehensively consequences are represented by an evaluation but is also a key to determining the type of analysis. Chapter 1 outlined factors that determined whether to conduct a CCA, CMA, CEA, CUA, or CBA.

Specify the options for comparison

As time and money for evaluation are limited, and because health services are complex and data on effectiveness of interventions limited, you often have to choose comparators from a wide range of possibilities. The choice of comparators has a fundamental impact on the type of evaluation conducted, approach to data collection and interpretation of findings (Cantor and Ganiats 1999). Table 2.1 summarizes the principal types of comparison options.

Table 2.1 Potential range of options against which to compare interventions

1 Current practice
a Single principal type(s) of intervention
b Mix of interventions
2 Best available alternative (e.g. as represented by clinical guidelines or low-cost alternative)
3 Do nothing
a Without the new intervention
b Without any care
PLUS …
4 Alternative levels of intensity for the new intervention

Source: Adapted from Cantor and Ganiats (1999)

As decisions about which services to provide are made in the context of what currently happens, the most relevant comparison for new interventions is usually current practice. However, current practice is not always easy to define because it usually consists of many different practices. Therefore, in defining current practice, one option is to choose the most frequently used intervention for comparison with the new intervention or alternatively to use several types of care as single comparators for the new treatment. The more types of current practice selected, the more data required and the more complex the analysis. In addition, defining current practice in this way would assume that each patient faces each type of care as a real option, which may not be the case if some patients are not eligible for some treatments. Therefore, a second possibility is to evaluate the mix of current treatments as a 'package'. However, effectiveness data are not always available for combinations of treatment.

Activity 2.1

In the previous paragraph, two main options were given for using current treatment as a comparator (one or more of the most frequently used treatments or a package of current treatment options). In Chapter 1 you learnt about incremental analysis. Using both pieces of knowledge, show how the choice of comparator would affect the specification of a study question.

 Feedback

Option 1: 'Assuming that patients could receive any of the (specified) current services or new treatment, which would be the most . . . cost-effective?'

Option 2: 'What is the incremental cost-effectiveness of moving from current practice to the new intervention?'

A second issue to consider is that current practice may itself not be efficient (Hutubessy *et al.* 2002) so that almost any comparison will appear efficient. In this situation you might choose the best available option (see Table 2.1) or a do nothing option. Two types of 'do nothing' option have been proposed: one that defines do nothing in terms of not doing the proposed intervention (Torrance *et al.* 1996); and another that uses no care at all (Hutubessy *et al.* 2002). Both are likely to have associated costs and impacts and you should not assume zero costs or effects. Whilst the first option is more relevant to current decision-making and less data intensive, the latter approach should be better for assessing efficiency in the long run and across health systems.

If a new intervention could be run at different levels of intensity (e.g. different frequencies or using different inclusion criteria) these alternatives should be added to the range of comparators considered. Once the options are selected for comparison, the description of each should be set out as for the new intervention and the questions identified above addressed.

Target population (noting spillover effects)

The target population is the group for whom the intervention is intended. It can vary by age, sex, disease and geography, and has a major impact on cost effectiveness. It is also important to identify whether there are subgroups for which separate analysis should be undertaken, such as for different age or ethnic groups. For example, one age-group of patients may use more or less resources and have a higher or lower effectiveness following an intervention. Alternatively, patients with particular symptoms may value changes in health very differently.

Activity 2.2

The extract below by Walker *et al.* (2002) describes a programme to train village health workers. Having read it, consider how you would frame an economic evaluation by addressing the questions and tasks below.

1 Which intervention options could be evaluated? (make sure you capture all parts of the options).
2 Identify who, does what, to whom, where, how often and with what results for the basic life skills training etc. option.
3 Select current practice as the comparator, define it and identify who, does what, to whom, where, how often and with what results.
4 Complete Table 2.2. This table has a standard set of issues (in the first column) that have to be considered at the start of any evaluation. It asks you to note down (in the second column) the options that you could choose from, for each issue. As choices of what to do and what to include in an economic evaluation always have to be made, you are asked to select one of the options identified (in the third column) and justify your choice (in the fourth column).
5 The tasks so far have taken you through parts of the intervention and options for comparison. Write down the full evaluative question that you think should be addressed.

Table 2.2 Drawing up the boundaries for analysis

Issues for consideration	Range of options that could be considered	Which approach will you use?	Justify your choice(s) here
Objectives of analysis			
Audience			
Viewpoint			
Time:			
a) Time of intervention			
b) Time over which benefits experienced			
c) Analytic horizon			
Which alternatives to the intervention could be used for comparison?			
Target population(s)			
Type of analysis			

Training village health workers

Pre-service training programmes based in nursing schools were developed in order to train a large number of village midwives (VMWs) in a relatively short period. The first of 60 000 trained VMWs were deployed in 1994. However, the quality of training was compromised by the need to place VMWs in villages as quickly as possible, and the midwives had little practical experience in conducting deliveries. The need for further in-service training and continuing education was recognized, and short courses were developed centrally and offered at district level. However . . . there were too many participants and too little hands-on care was given. Those responsible for the training of VMWs were, and still are, facility-based midwives (FMWs, known locally as *bidan*). The pressure of in-service training duties has made it impossible to update the training of the FMWs through refresher courses.

. . . programmes intended to improve the knowledge and skills of FMWs and VMWs in the province of South Kalimantan were conducted during 1995–98. They were designed and implemented through a partnership that included the national and provincial levels of the Ministry of Health, the Indonesian Midwifery Association and the MotherCare/John Snow Inc. Project, funded by the United States Agency for International Development. Technical assistance was provided by the American College of Nurse Midwives through the MotherCare Project . . .

Activities began in 1995 in three districts of South Kalimantan, namely Banjar, Barito Kuala, and Hulu Sungai Selatan. Training in life-saving skills (LSS), developed by the American College of Nurse Midwives, was adapted to meet the needs of the midwives and the community, as determined by a training needs assessment conducted in November 1995. It was necessary for the FMWs and VMWs to improve their capabilities in the handling of obstetric emergencies and in the normal aspects of antenatal, labour delivery and postpartum care. A manual was developed to meet the needs of both groups. The training for FMWs became known as advanced LSS and that for VMWs as basic LSS.

Two hospitals were established during 1996 as training centres on the basis of their capacity to support competence-based training, particularly the availability of adequate clinical experience for each participant (15 deliveries per participant per month). A third training centre was established at another hospital in March 1998. Each hospital underwent a one-week site preparation during which the programmes were introduced and all staff working in antenatal, delivery and postpartum wards received training to encourage the staff at the training centres to apply the same skills and techniques taught in LSS.

Eighteen FMWs were selected as trainers and attended: a two-week course on clinical skills in advanced LSS; a separate clinical training-of-trainers course for the basic LSS course; and a one-week course for teaching skills.

An integrated system was developed to support the initial in-service training through regular peer review visits by trained FMWs and incorporation of the aggregated information from these visits into continuing education sessions. All LSS-trained FMWs were trained as peer reviewers and were expected to make annual visits to each other and to VMWs who received in-service education.

↻ **Feedback**

1 The two different parts of the intervention (which could be evaluated separately or together as a combined programme) are:

    a) advanced life-saving skills training, peer review visits and continuing education for facility-based midwives;

    b) basic life-saving skills training, peer review visits and continuing education for village-based midwives.

2 See Table 2.3 for description of option 1b above.

3 See Table 2.3. Note for this example, the selected current practice was the government-trained *bidan* who had not participated in any MotherCare training programme.

Table 2.3 Description of alternatives for evaluation

	Option 1 (intervention)	Option 2 (comparator)
Who?	FMWs who had received 2 weeks additional training in advanced life saving skills and training skills	FMWs
Does what?	1) Basic training using a locally adapted course based from American College of Nurse Midwives. 2) Equips VMWs at the end of the training period. 3) Regular visits to review practice of newly trained VMWs	Additional refresher training courses
To whom?	VMWs	VMWs
Where?	1) Hospital based training site. 2) Visits to villages to observe VMWs	'Offered at district level' (in hospital)
How often?	1) Initial training received once for five days. 2) Peer review four times per year per VMW	It looks like a policy of short courses exists in theory but not in practice 'due to the pressure of in-service training'
What are the results?	1) Improved knowledge on life-saving skills. 2) Changed delivery and referral practices. 3) improved health of mother and babies	The objectives should be the same as the intervention

4 See Table 2.4 (opposite).

5 'From the viewpoint of health providers and consumers, what is the cost-effectiveness of the package of MotherCare training in the three districts in South Kalimantan compared with the level of training usually offered by the Ministry of Health?' The combined package is recommended as it is likely to be difficult to attribute impact on morbidity to a specific part of the package.

Table 2.4 Drawing up the boundaries for analysis

Issues for consideration	Range of options that could be considered	Approach chosen	Justification of choice
Objectives of analysis	a) Continue to provide the new programme in same district. b) Adding or replacing the new programme in other district(s)	First a) and then b)	a) Is based on evidence from the locality and b) will require more of a 'what if' approach
Audience	Ministry of Health (central and district), MotherCare, Indonesian Midwifery Association, USAID, John Snow Inc.	MoH and John Snow Inc.	John Snow Inc. was funding research and trying to influence the MoH and USAID
Viewpoint	Government, patients and families, health providers, MotherCare, society	Health providers and patients/ families	This would have to be the MoH position if MotherCare project ended as expected
Time	a) From set-up to covering all current VMW (could also account for attrition rate of VMWs). Could consider running for 1 to × years. b) Will depend on benefit measure. If there is a mortality impact then take lifetime of babies. c) Maximum of a & b	From inception to end of programme (1995–8)	This captured all costs and effectiveness was limited to intermediate indicators (of changed knowledge) rather than impact on morbidity or mortality
Alternatives comparison?	Each part of the intervention could be a comparator as well as existing practice	Existing practice	Would represent the incremental change experienced for costs and effects
Target population(s)	For training, all FMWs and VMWs expected to be in post in a given time period. For effectiveness, it is pregnant women and their newborns	MFWs and VMWs	Because no data on impact on women or babies available
Type of analysis	CEA, CUA, CBA, CCA	CEA	Evaluation only funded costing not transfer of effects into utility weights or money values

Summary

You have learnt how to frame an economic evaluation taking into account: the objectives of the analysis; the audience; the perspective of the analysis; the analytic horizon; the specifics of the interventions being compared; and the target population. You will now learn about the role of decision analysis.

References

Cantor SB and Ganiats TG (1999) Incremental cost-effectiveness analysis: the optimal strategy depends on the strategy set. *Journal of Clinical Epidemiology* 52(6):517–22.

Drummond MF, O'Brien B, Stoddart GL and Torrance GW (1997) *Methods for the economic evaluation of health care programmes*. Oxford: Oxford Medical Publications.

Gold MR, Siegel JE, Russell LB and Weinstein MC (eds) (1996) *Cost-effectiveness in health and medicine*. Oxford: Oxford University Press.

Hill SR, Mitchell AS and Henry DA (2000) Problems with the interpretation of pharmacoeconomic analyses: a review of submissions to the Australian Pharmaceutical Benefits Scheme. *Journal of the American Medical Association* 283(16):2116–21.

Hutubessy RC, Baltussen RM, Torres-Edejer TT and Evans DB (2002) Generalised cost-effectiveness analysis: an aid to decision making in health. *Applied Health Economics and Policy* 1(2): 89–95.

Torrance GW, Siegel JE and Luce BR (1996) Chapter 2: Framing and designing the cost-effectiveness analysis, in M. Gold *et al.* (eds) *Cost-effectiveness in health and medicine*. Oxford: Oxford University Press.

Walker D and Fox-Rushby JA (2000) Critical review of economic evaluations of communicable disease interventions in developing countries. *Health Economics* 9(8): 681–98.

Walker D, McDermott J, Fox-Rushby J, Nadjib M, Widiatmoko D, Tanjung M and Achadi E (2002) Cost, effects and cost-effectiveness of midwifery training in South Kalimantan, Indonesia. *Bulletin of the World Health Organization* 80(1): 47–55.

Further reading

Farnham PG, Ackerman SP and Haddix AC (1996) Chapter 2: Study design, in A Haddix *et al.* (eds) *Prevention effectiveness: a guide to decision analysis and economic evaluation*. Oxford: Oxford University Press.

3 | The role of decision analysis in economic evaluation

Overview

Economic evaluation aims to help select, from at least two health care interventions, the best option. This can be a complex decision based on a variety of data. Decision analysis is a useful framework on which to build economic evaluations. It not only helps structure the problem but also guides the use and interpretation of data. However, this is not the only approach to decision-making within the health sector: 'evidence based medicine', based on the systematic review of clinical evidence, has developed rapidly since the mid 1990s. In this chapter you will learn about evidence-based medicine and contrast it with decision analysis. You will also learn how to justify the use of decision analysis in economic evaluation as well as in medical decision-making.

Learning objectives

After working through this chapter, you will be able to:

- distinguish between alternative approaches to decision analysis
- recognize the importance of decision analysis for structuring decisions about selecting the best options for care (at an individual and policy level)

Key terms

Clinical or professional judgement The decision taken by a clinician as to whether or not a patient has a normative need.

Decision analysis This approach aims to identify all relevant choices for a specific decision and to quantify the relative expected benefits (or costs) of each option. The range of choices can be represented in a decision tree.

Evidence-based medicine Movement within medicine and related professions to base clinical practice on the most rigorous scientific basis, principally informed by the results of randomized controlled trials of effectiveness of interventions.

Health technology assessment Systematic reviewing of existing evidence and providing an evaluation of the effectiveness, cost-effectiveness and impact, both on patient health and on the health care system, of medical technology and its use.

Meta-analysis An overview of all the valid research evidence. If feasible, the quantitative results of different studies may be combined to obtain an overall result, referred to as a 'statistical meta-analysis'.

> **Modelling** Simplifying reality and synthesizing data to capture the consequences of different decision options. This might involve simulating an event or a patient's or population's life experience mathematically.

Introduction

Decision analysis is an approach used to help formulate questions and to quantify the relative value of each option evaluated. It is one of several decision-making approaches used in choosing therapies for individual patients as well as in public policy. It can underpin and complement other approaches. In this chapter you will compare decision analytic approaches with 'evidence-based medicine' (EBM) and work towards a conclusion that decision analysis is appropriate but that some of the approaches used within EBM can be used within a decision analytic structure. The chapter ends by considering whether and how decision analysis is used.

 Activity 3.1

The following extract by Jack Dowie (1996) describes developments in the application of research evidence in medical decision-making and discusses their potential and their limitations. He introduces the concept of decision analysis based medical decision-making (DABMDM). As you read the extract, make notes to answer the following questions:

1 In your opinion, what approaches (other than decision analysis) are used to make decisions about which therapies should be selected?
2 What are the main differences between decision analysis and EBM?
3 What are the advantages of decision analysis over EBM?
4 What do you think are likely to be the challenges of introducing decision analysis into patient care and public policy?

 Decision analysis for medical decision-making

Introduction

Three broad movements are currently seeking to change the world of medicine . . .

1 The proponents of EBM are mainly concerned with ensuring strategies of proven clinical effectiveness are adopted.
2 Health economists are mainly concerned to establish that cost-effectiveness and not clinical effectiveness is the criterion used on determining option selection.
3 A variety of patient support and public interest groups, including many health economists, are mainly concerned with ensuring that patient and public preferences drive clinical and policy decisions.

It is the thesis of this paper that all three movements will experience continuing disappointment and frustration until they recognise the need for a paradigmatic shift in ways of thinking, judging and deciding at all levels of the health care system, including clinical practice . . .

Alternative paradigms

An important feature of the current paradigm is encapsulated in the holistic use of the term 'medicine'. As used in phrases such as 'practising medicine' (evidence based or not), it serves the discursive purpose of confounding two conceptually distinct activities: the making of decisions and the carrying out of actions (actions which may or may not constitute the implementation of an immediately preceding decision) . . .

. . . Within a paradigm that fails to stress the distinction between deciding and doing it is not at all surprising that 'facts' and 'value judgments' (including those about costs) are left to contaminate each other in unknown ways during the practice of medicine, rather than being analysed separately and integrated – as they must be in order to arrive at a choice – in a clear and defensible manner.

There is, therefore, one overwhelmingly important procedural reason why the existing paradigm cannot and should not survive much longer. Decision owners – patients, groups and communities – cannot play their proper role in decision making unless 'deciding' is separated from 'doing' and unless this separation is done in such a way as to make it possible for knowledge values and costs to be clearly separated at all times prior to their necessary integration in choice . . .

It follows that the change required is one which replaces the holistic paradigm, with its confounding and confusions, by one in which the two fundamental dualities are not merely accepted and acknowledged in hand-waving fashion but are constantly stressed and placed at the heart of all professional training, practice and policy making. Firstly, medicine is a dual activity, in which decision making must be clearly distinguished from acting. Competence in deciding, in conjunction with decision owners, whether to order a test for or operate on a patient has no necessary association with competence in administering the test, describing the test results, or carrying out the operation. Consequently, the existence of skills in decision making per se must be recognised in all curricula, appointments and institutional arrangements and a high correlation in competence in the two activities not assumed. Secondly, medical decision making always involves processing two distinct components and it is vital that values are accorded at least equal importance with knowledge of the facts (which is often partial and probabilistic).

. . . The key to the new paradigm lies not simply in the centrality assigned to the distinction between deciding and doing, but in the demand that deciding – and hence the doing – be based on a much greater degree of formal analysis than at present. Only by raising the analytical level of medical decision making can the necessary separation of facts and values/costs be achieved and ensured.

It is not, of course, intended in any way to imply that there is no formal analysis undertaken in medicine at the moment, only that the amount is relatively low compared to what would occur in the new paradigm and, much more importantly, that most of it is not decision analysis . . .

. . . Classical decision analysis is, in my view, the only form of analysis that provides for the separation of facts, values and costs and for the integration of all the elements of a decision in a clearly specified and rationally defensible manner . . . Modelling within a decision analytic framework not only ensures that all the evidence needed for a decision can be systematically identified, but also that, when collected and critiqued, this evidence will be integrated in a systematic and transparent way into the decision. The robustness of the conclusion reached in the decision analysis can be assessed under varying assumptions as to the quality of each piece of evidence and the agreements and disagreements of various parties to the decision precisely located. Decision analysis can, therefore, make particularly strong claims as a decision making procedure, apart from its ability to identify the optimal course of action under specific assumptions . . . Like any tool it has the potential to be hijacked by one interest to oppress others. But its explicitness and transparency compared with either current procedures or alternative techniques will minimise the chances of such attempts at abuse being successful at the same time they deter attempts to avoid necessary trade-offs in the pursuit of unattainable ideas.

EBM, DABMDM and current practice

. . . Currently, practitioners faced with explaining the impact of a piece of evidence on their decision will usually be found saying that they 'took it into account and bore it in mind', or words to that effect. The precise implications of 'taking into account and bearing in mind' are unknown to most who engage in them and are certainly not explicable to others . . . it is taken for granted that we will be reassured by the statement that 'The evidence will not automatically dictate patient care but will provide the factual basis on which decision can be made, taking all aspects of patient care into consideration'. What this really means is that the rigour of EBM is to vanish as soon as we have documented the 'clinical facts', to be replaced by the 'clinical judgement' process and, one fears in many cases, the power-based inequalities of clinical teams . . .

. . . As far as decision making is concerned, there is never any doubt that at the end of the day practitioners are going to discuss and critique the evidence gathered (including that provided by any decision analysis turned up in the literature) and 'take everything into consideration', 'bearing everything in mind' . . .

. . . The concern here, therefore, is with the level of analysis that characterises the overarching decision making process (clinical or managerial), within which (1) a problem is framed and particular evidence is deemed to be relevant, necessary or desirable, (2) the evidence is sought and evaluated, and (3) the evidence obtained – full, partial or none – is integrated into an assessment that determines choice of action. That a great deal of high level analysis can go on in the middle phase is not disputed. It is the analytical level of the before and after phases – stages 1 and 4 . . . that is at issue (Table 3.1).

Table 3.1 EBM process

The practice of EBM is a process of lifelong, problem-based learning in which caring for our patients creates the need for evidence about diagnosis, prognosis, therapy, and other clinical and health care issues. In the EBM process we:
1 Convert these information needs into answerable questions.
2 Track down, with maximum efficiency, the best evidence with which to answer them (whether from the clinical examination, the diagnostic laboratory, the published literature, or other sources).
3 Critically appraise that evidence for its validity (closeness to the truth) and usefulness (clinical applicability).
4 Apply the results of this appraisal in our clinical practice; and
5 Evaluate our performance.

Source: Dowie (1996)

It is clear that for proponents of EBM the overarching decision making process is not itself to be aided or guided by formal, explicit and comprehensive modelling and structuring. But such modelling and structuring (Table 3.2) is essential to ensure that:

1   The necessary search for evidence is guided by the requisites of the decision as a whole and not by a partial formulation of the problem or problems within it.

2 The cognitive limitations or practitioners, along with all other human beings, do not lead to errors of distortions in the application of the evidence yielded by their searches to the case in hand.

3 The integration of all component pieces of evidence into a choice is done transparently as well as systematically – and hence equitably, in that every individual in the decision making group, including both professional and lay persons, can and must make explicit the factual and the value bases if their conclusion or recommendation . . .

Table 3.2 Six steps in DABMDM

1. Model the presenting or current patient case in decision analytic form, carefully separating and defining possible actions (options), 'knowledge' (certainties and uncertainties), possible outcomes, outcome valuations and costs.
2. Search the literature for relevant articles and consult relevant colleagues to check that the modelling is sound and to establish baselines values and sensitivity ranges for the probabilities, utilities and costs required.
3. Consult patients to elicit their preferences – to be constructed if they do not pre-exist – and hence utility values.
4. Evaluate the model to determine the optimal strategy under various conditions.
5. If alternative models of decision making are brought into the discussion, engage in comparative evaluation of the decision analytic modelling of the problem and its implications, ensuring that the alternative models are exposed to equally stringent critiquing regarding both the inputs on which they are based and the way their component inputs are integrated into a choice.
6. Consult the patient and implement or iterate from the appropriate step above.

Note: steps 1 and 2 may be bypassed in whole or in part if a decision analysis for the presenting or currently condition is already available on-line. Including costs is not a central difference to EBM and DABMDM
Source: Dowie (1996)

Why DABMDM is a pre-requisite for cost-effective and preference based medicine

. . . To economists it is simply ludicrous to suggest that a group of people could sit around examining evidence relating to the costs and likely outcomes of various options, on the one hand, and evidence relating to patient or public preferences on the other, and informally – without the aid of a well-specified model on paper or screen – arrive at a verdict as to which is the optimal strategy. They wouldn't do it and wouldn't try. This isn't because, compared with clinicians and other medical decision makers, they are particularly stupid or inexpert or lack years of experience. It is because they know that, being human, they don't have the computational capabilities to undertake this task satisfactorily unaided and in an unstructured manner. And neither do doctors.

◯⤸ **Feedback**

1 There is a range of potential approaches. You may have come across the first two in your own experience and the others if you have read more widely:

 a) personal views of doctor (clinical judgement), patient and/or researchers who 'take account of' evidence or values
 b) historical (e.g. continue what was done last year) or political approach
 c) needs assessment or estimating the burden of disease; this approach accounts for the size of a problem and sometimes the cost but not the expected benefits (e.g. Murray and Lopez 1996)

d) programme budgeting and marginal analysis; this is a pragmatic approach to decision-making based on opportunity costs and changes 'at the margin' (Mitton and Donaldson 2004)

e) focus on 'core' or 'essential' services – however, Eddy (1991) points out the difficulties of defining what is essential and who should decide and argues for clarifying costs, benefits and harms and including patient views.

2 EBM vs DABMDM:

a) EBM is problem-focused whereas DABMDM is decision-focused.

b) most work in EBM occurs in stages 2 and 3 whereas in DABMDM places greater emphasis on stage I (Tables 3.I and 3.2)

c) EBM does not specifically mention incorporating patient values or costs and more emphasis is placed on clinical issues.

d) further reading of the paper highlights the focus of EBM on randomized trials even given difficulties of generalizing results to other settings.

3 Advantages of DABMDM:

a) decisions can be structured in a more accountable way and assumptions tested

b) more targeted at answering policy-relevant questions

c) more inclusive of other policy-relevant data (costs, preferences of different groups)

d) better able to handle a larger body of data within a decision.

4 Challenges:

a) Some general problems might include: access to computers; data entry to models may be tedious (and the more complex the model the greater the data requirements and ensuing tedium); difficulties in conveying the subtlety of clinical information to a programme; not all practitioners will have the necessary knowledge of databases; difficulties in interpreting and communicating results to patients; cost of developing and managing decision support systems

b) Finding out about patients' values will take doctors time to do; patients may or may not want to give their own values and finding out may itself be stressful for patients who are already sick – you may think of other issues too

c) in public policy, simple models may be easier to explain to decision-makers but lack sufficient reality whereas complex models may take too long to explain, increase uncertainties and require more data – You may think of other issues too.

Is decision analysis being used today?

Decision analytic modelling has increased exponentially in recent years. Between 1992 and 1996, 32% of economic evaluations for drugs consisted of decision analytic models whereas between 1997 and 2001 the percentage had increased to 42% (OHE HEED 2004). Modelling appears to be used differentially depending on the type of economic evaluation. For example, Nixon *et al.* (2000) found that models were used in 16.7% of CEAs and in 20% of CBAs but in 60.2% in CUAs. Perhaps these results are not surprising given that in practice CUAs are often based on literature reviews.

In high-income countries, modelling has been linked to the growing field of health technology assessment and the development of a number of national agencies developing guidance on best practice for pharmaceutical and other health technologies. Decision analytic techniques have been used with economic evaluation in a wide variety of cases, from options for case management with anti-retrovirals to approaches to improving links between primary and secondary care for childbirth. It has been particularly useful when a health care intervention has impacts over long periods of time or long lags in impact such that effects are unlikely to be observed in randomized trials (Chilcott *et al.* 2003). In low-income countries, there has been less use of decision analysis alongside economic evaluation but it is increasing, helped by a few high-profile examples (e.g. Goldie *et al.* 2001).

There are now several guides to good practice in undertaking decision analytic modelling. Philips *et al.* (2004) reviewed and synthesized all good practice guidelines and provided guidance for developing better quality models that can be justified, are accessible to review and are relevant to decision-makers.

Most recently, decision analytic modelling has been linked to producing research findings more efficiently using 'expected value of information' analysis. This type of analysis is related to reducing decision-makers' uncertainty. It can also help in determining the size and length of randomized trials.

Summary

You have learnt about the different approaches to decision analysis and its importance for structuring decisions. You went on to consider the limitations of evidence-based medicine and the need to incorporate information on patients' values and on costs. You will now go on to learn about one approach to decision analysis – the use of decision trees.

References

Chilcott J, Brennan A, Booth A, Karnon J and Tappenden P (2003) The role of modelling in prioritising and planning clinical trials. *Health Technology Assessment* 7:23, www.ncchta. org/fullmono/mon723.pdf.

Dowie J (1996) 'Evidence-based', 'cost-effective' and 'preference-driven' medicine: decision analysis based medical decision making is the pre-requisite. *Journal of Health Services Research & Policy* 1(2):104–12.

Eddy DM (1991) What care is 'essential'? What services are 'basic'? *Journal of the American Medical Association* 265(6):782, 786–8.

Goldie SJ, Kuhn L, Denny L, Pollack A and Wright TC (2001) Policy analysis of cervical cancer screening strategies in low-resource settings: clinical benefits and cost-effectiveness. *Journal of the American Medical Association*, 285(24):3107–15. Erratum in: *Journal of the American Medical Association* 2001 286(9):1026.

Mitton C and Donaldson C (2004) Health care priority setting: principles, practice and challenges. *Cost Effectiveness and Resource Allocation* 2:3, free web access through www.resource-allocation.com/content/2/1/3.

Murray CJL and Lopez AD (eds) (1996) *The global burden of disease*. Cambridge, MA: Harvard University Press.

Nixon J, Stoykova B, Glanville J, Christie J, Drummond M and Kleinjen J (2000) The UK NHS

Economic Evaluation Database. *International Journal of Technology Assessment in Health Care*, 16(3):731–42.

OHE HEED (2004) Briefing Paper No. 40, March. London: Office of Health Economics.

Philips Z, Ginnelly L, Sculpher M, Claxton K, Golder S, Riemsma R, Woolacoot N and Glanville J (2004) Review of guidelines for good practice in decision-analytic modelling in health technology assessment. *Health Technology Assessment* 8(36):iii–iv, ix–xi, 1–158, www.ncchta.org/execsumm/summ836.htm.

Further reading

Claxton K, Ginnelly L, Sculpher M, Philips Z and Palmer S (2004) A pilot study on the use of decision theory and value of information analysis as part of the NHS Health Technology Assessment programme. *Health Technology Assessment* 8(31), www.ncchta.org/execsumm/summ831.htm.

Jack Dowie has written several papers on the role of decision-making in health care and these can currently be accessed on www.lshtm.ac.uk/pehru/staff/jdowie.html.

Ginnelly L and Manca A (2003) The use of decision models in mental health economic evaluation: challenges and opportunities. *Applied Health Economics and Health Policy* 2(3):157–64.

Good journal papers on this subject appear in *Medical Decision Making*. To download papers free, go to http://mdm.sagepub.com/archive/.

4   Introduction to economic modelling

Overview

In this chapter you will learn about the use of modelling in decision-making and work through the design of a decision tree for assessing the most (cost-) effective policy option. You will learn how to: define problems; set up model structures; assign and apply probabilities; assign values (costs and effectiveness) to consequences; calculate expected values for treatment options and interpret the results.

Learning objectives

After working through this chapter, you will be able to:

- understand the basic applications of modelling in decision-making in public health
- construct a simple decision tree
- populate the decision tree with data by assigning probabilities and values to costs and benefits
- average out and fold back to calculate the expected value of competing policy options
- discuss the advantages and disadvantages of using decision analysis in public health

Key terms

Chance node The point in a decision tree where an outcome is subject to chance and to which a probability can be attached.

Decision node The point in a decision tree where a decision must be made between competing and mutually exclusive policy or treatment options.

Parameter An input to a model.

Pay-off Denotes the net value of the specific outcome represented by terminal node.

Terminal node The end-point of a branch in a decision tree, where final outcomes for that path are defined.

Utility values Numerical representation of the degree of satisfaction with health status, health outcome or health care.

Introduction

The aim of decision analysis is to make explicit the best decision (from at least two options) at the time a decision is made, given available information as well as the values and logic that apply to the decision. Figure 4.1 shows the range of information that might be used to construct a model. It shows the types of information for each option used as inputs to a model in order to predict the output, in this example an ICER.

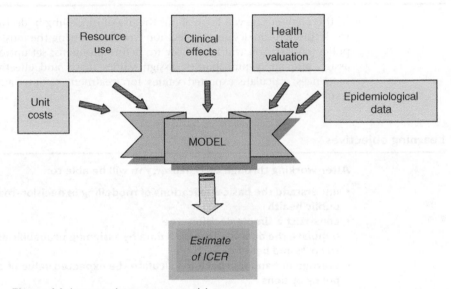

Figure 4.1 Inputs and outputs to a model

A model is a simplification of the real world, with only the most important components considered. A good model enables you to work out what is likely to happen if you make particular decisions. Modelling encourages decision-making to be explicit and can comprehensively deal with the inputs and outcomes of decision options. In addition, it can help identify gaps in current evidence. Models are statistically attractive as they allow a range of uncertainties to be reflected and statistical testing of hypotheses. Economic modelling techniques are increasingly used in making local and national health care decisions, especially in high income countries. For example, the Pharmaceutical Benefits Advisory Committee in Australia use economic modelling when deciding which pharmaceuticals should be publicly paid for in the Australian health system.

Modelling can be useful in several situations:

- when an important decision needs to be made in the absence of clear direction from the data;
- for extrapolating beyond the data observed in a randomized trial;
- for linking intermediate clinical end-points to final outcomes (such as linking bone mineral density and long-term risk of bone fractures);
- for generalizing results to other settings;

- for synthesizing head-to-head comparisons where relevant randomized trials don't exist;
- to indicate the need for further research.

Activity 4.1

Think of circumstances, for each of the reasons given above, for modelling.

Feedback

- If adopting an intervention implies very high future costs, decision-makers are more likely to want a model. This happened with the UK heart transplantation programme in the 1980s.
- The incidence of pneumonia due to haemophilus influenza is often not known (even if the number of pneumonia cases in hospital is) but decisions are still taken on whether to adopt the relevant vaccine or not.
- Randomized trials often only measure short-term or intermediate outcomes but economic models often need data for a lifetime.
- Trials may be limited to clinical end-points (Chapters 11 and 12) but an economic evaluation may require calculation of QALYs.
- Wanting to predict results from a trial to routine practice or from one country to another.
- Where trials have not used a relevant comparator. This can happen when data from one country uses different treatments in current practice or because a do-nothing option is used.
- Calculating the expected value of perfect information can indicate which parts of the model most reduce the uncertainty in outcomes (Claxton and Posnett 1996).

A good model should reflect current clinical practice and therefore use an appropriate comparator. It should be based on the best quality data available (possibly a meta-analysis of existing studies). The model needs to cover (be 'run' for) an appropriate time period. For example, when evaluating a lipid-lowering drug, the long-term benefits (such as reduction in stroke risk) may not be evident for many years. To capture all relevant costs and benefits, the model should be run for many years. However, when evaluating a new drug for a fatal condition (such as some types of cancer), the model can be run for a shorter period since the life expectancy of the cohort will be low. It is also important to explore the uncertainty of data inputs and model structure using sensitivity analysis (which you will learn more about in Chapters 14 and 15).

A key characteristic of all models should be their transparency and reproducibility so that the validity of the model and its results can be checked. It is essential that a model has high internal and external validity. Agencies such as INFARMED (part of the Ministry of Health) in Portugal and combinations of agencies (e.g. the 'economic', 'market approval' and 'transparency' committees in France) consider different economic models submitted by various stakeholders (including pharmaceutical companies) prior to making policy recommendations on the reimbursement of health services or proposals to cut costs. These agencies have set up extensive review processes to check the validity of models, as models submitted by different stakeholders may disagree.

The modelling process can be time-consuming, complex and is often beyond the technical reach of those making decisions. It can be difficult for decision-makers to know to what extent the model incorporates all the factors they would wish to be included. Changes in clinical practice can lead to the underlying assumptions, parameters, and comparators becoming inappropriate in a short space of time. While changes in parameter values can easily be accounted for in an existing model, once the comparators change the structure of a model may need to change.

The two most common types of model are decision trees and Markov models (you will learn about the latter in Chapter 7). A decision tree is a flow diagram showing the logical structure of the problem. The term 'decision tree' is used because options are arranged to resemble a tree in appearance. They are particularly suited to decisions about acute care, diseases that occur once only, and decisions with short time frames (e.g. a short-term screening decision).

The basic steps in constructing a decision tree are:

- scoping the research question;
- constructing a decision tree;
- estimating probabilities;
- assigning values to consequences (for costs and outcomes);
- averaging out and folding back to estimate expected values and summary measures;
- testing results by using sensitivity analysis.

Scoping the research question

Before starting to build the decision tree, the problem that needs to be addressed should be defined clearly. This requires considering the same issues covered in Chapter 3. The question needs to be specified in a way that allows the best available data to be used. If it becomes a very broad question there is unlikely to be enough information or the task may get unmanageable. However, if defined very narrowly it may no longer be applicable to the population for which the decision is being made.

Decision trees depend on the boundaries set for the analysis (e.g. the definition of the population or the clinical indication). It is important that options must be distinct and not overlap and that branches emanating from a decision node represent all the options including the current care. Experienced clinicians, researchers with an expertise in the field, patients, and professional and lay carers should accept the model structure.

Constructing a decision tree

A decision option is defined as a possible choice among all options. Each possible choice that is included in the decision analysis is called a decision option. One of

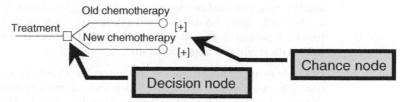

Figure 4.2 Treatment options, decision node and chance node

these will be current practice. A decision node (usually drawn as a square) represents the first point of choice in the decision tree. Decision trees are conventionally written from left to right, starting with the initial decision node on the extreme left and moving to the final outcomes on the extreme right. Figure 4.2 presents the first step in constructing a tree. The sequence of chance nodes from left to right in the decision tree usually follows the sequence of events over time. A line attached to the box represents each decision option. If there is a [+] sign at the end of the node, it usually means that there is more to come beyond that point in the tree.

In economic evaluation it is standard practice to compare new treatments with current practice. As you learnt in Chapter 2, choice of the comparator is crucial. It is important to note that the comparator does not need to be the gold-standard treatment. As economic evaluations are often designed to evaluate a new treatment to replace an existing one, the comparator should be chosen as the treatment which is the most commonly used in current practice.

Figure 4.2 shows the comparison of two treatment options for an old versus new chemotherapy drug (for treatment of cancer). Once the comparators are selected, any events that follow happen with probabilities – they are 'chance' events. Outcomes that are not under the control of decision-makers are denoted by a chance node (symbolized by a circle). A decision tree may compare more than two options and may also compare very different options.

Each outcome from a chance event is labelled and denoted by a line attached to the circle. Figure 4.3 shows that the first outcome of having the 'Old chemotherapy' is the presence of haematological (blood related) side-effects or not. If someone does not have a side-effect, that is the end of outcomes associated with the treatment

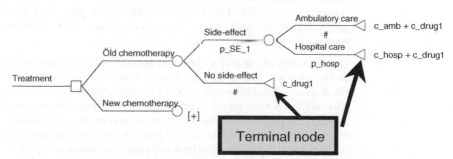

Figure 4.3 Development of the decision tree; chance events and terminal nodes

and this is represented by a terminal node (triangle). However, if a person does have a side-effect, Figure 4.3 shows that the outcome would be to receive either ambulatory or inpatient (hospital) care (after which terminal nodes indicate the end of information relevant to the decision).

One rule is important to note at this stage: the events at a chance node must be mutually exclusive and exhaustive. Therefore, all possible events must be listed and there must be no overlap in the definition of these events. This also means that the sum of the probabilities stemming from each individual chance node before any other node must sum to 1.0. For example, in Figure 4.3, the probability of a side-effect occurring is indicated by 'p_SE_1'. Therefore, the probability of side-effects not occurring is 1 – 'p_SE_1' (denoted by #).

 Activity 4.2

In Figure 4.3, what impact would different time frames have on the structure of the model and the data required? What would an appropriate time frame be?

 Feedback

The time frame selected would affect how many events could occur and this would affect the number of chance nodes if each time period (lets say a year) had different probabilities for events to occur. Where probabilities are constant each year, it would not affect the number of chance nodes but may affect the value of probabilities. The time frame would also affect the quantity of data required as well as costs and effects in the terminal node. The appropriate time frame should be one that accounts for all costs and outcomes. For example, if the modelling question is about a chronic disease (such as diabetes) where most of the clinical outcomes will occur five to ten years later, it would not be appropriate to run the model for one year only. However, if you are modelling a highly fatal disease where most patients die within a year, modelling beyond one year would not be needed.

Estimating probabilities

Once the basic structure of the decision tree has been set out, the next step is to 'populate the model'. This is split into two parts: providing an estimate of all the probabilities; and valuing any consequences for costs and outcomes at the end of each path or branch.

The reliability of estimates depends crucially on the quality of data and any biases in the data will bias a model's results. Some data are inherently more uncertain (such as anecdotal evidence, expert opinion or small non-randomized studies) and this can also lead to broader confidence intervals and more uncertain conclusions. In selecting probabilities for each part of the model, it is useful to note any variation for use later in the sensitivity analysis. As the sources of data for probabilities are also relevant to collecting cost and outcome data, a comparison of approaches is given in Chapter 6.

Modellers always need to consider their data sources carefully from the variety that exist. Therefore, Nuitjen (1999) recommends that all models should present information that allows readers to:

- understand the nature of the data sources;
- understand the methods and criteria used for the selection and use of data sources;
- evaluate the strengths, weaknesses and potential sources of bias; and
- judge whether the model uses data from a population to whom the results are expected to apply.

Assigning values to consequences (for costs and outcomes)

Once probabilities have been found for each chance node (or plausible assumptions made), values can be attached. It is very important to reference the sources of data and to explain any assumption in detail to ensure the transparency and the reproducibility of the results. Values are required for final benefits and for costs of events. In Figure 4.3 the average cost of ambulatory care and drugs was represented by 'c_amb + c_drug1' at the end of the first branch of the tree. Note that in this eventuality patients would incur both the cost of the ambulatory care and the cost of drugs (for simplicity, assume that full drug costs are incurred for all patients). Figure 4.4 lists the average cost per person for different aspects of care.

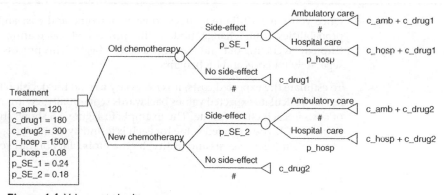

Figure 4.4 Values attached to costs

✎ Activity 4.3

Calculate the total cost of care per person for each terminal node (this assumes a person has all events in a specific branch of the tree).

↻ Feedback

$$c\_amb + c\_drug1 = £300$$

$$c\_hosp + c\_drug1 = £1680$$

$$c\_amb + c\_drug2 = £420$$

$$c\_hosp + c\_drug2 = £1800$$

$$c\_drug1 = £180$$

$$c\_drug2 = £300$$

To represent the value of benefits, a set of utility values might be applied. These could be as simple as 0 or 1 to represent being dead or alive but may also account for differences in quality of life. In Chapters 12 and 13 you will learn how this can be done and in Chapter 15 you will learn about what sources of data for utility values exist. Assume the following utility scores: 0.88 after ambulatory care; 0.65 after hospital care; and 0.99 when no side-effects are experienced. These values would be presented at the terminal nodes as appropriate.

Averaging out and folding back to estimate expected values and summary measures

Once you have attributed values to each outcome and cost and established the probabilities from chance nodes, the process of calculating expected values through 'averaging out and folding back' can begin. This process needs to happen separately for costs and for benefits.

To estimate the expected costs, it is necessary to read the decision tree from right to left and calculate expected values backwards sequentially, giving an expected value of costs at each chance node. The example in Figure 4.5 shows the expected value to be £410.4. The expected value for each is found by multiplying the consequence of the event (such as costs and utility) by the probability of the event occurring and

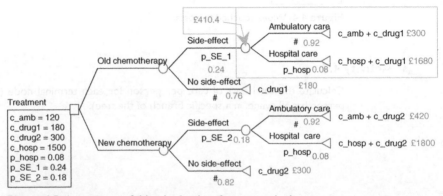

Figure 4.5 Averaging out folding back values for expected values

adding up these 'weighted' values at the chance node that led to the outcomes, i.e. (£300 × 0.92) + (£1680 × 0.08) = £410.40. The next step would be to read the decision tree one more branch to the left in order to calculate the expected cost of using the old chemotherapy. This time the calculation uses the expected cost of having a side-effect as £410.4 with the calculation for the expected cost of the old chemotherapy being (£410.4 × 0.24) + (£180 × 0.76) = £235. The calculation of expected utility values would happen in the same way but use the utility values instead of the costs.

 Activity 4.4

Using Figure 4.5, calculate the expected cost of the new chemotherapy and the expected utility of the old and new chemotherapies (the final utility scores were given after the feedback to Activity 4.3).

Feedback

The expected costs, shown below in Figure 4.6, indicate that 'Old chemotherapy' costs less at 235.30.

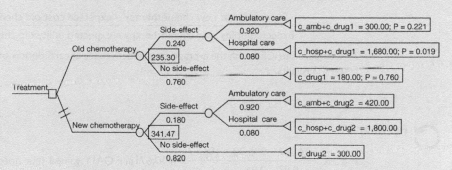

Note: The // across the first decision option indicates that this is not the best branch – it is broken (note that for utilities higher values are more desirable, whereas for costs the option with lower overall cost should be chosen).

Figure 4.6 Calculated costs

The expected utilities, shown in Figure 4.7, indicate that the 'New chemotherapy' option has a higher utility value of 0.97.

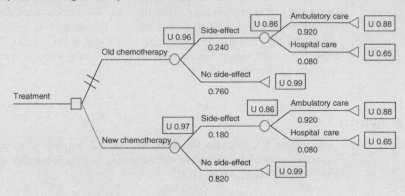

Figure 4.7 Expected utilities

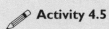 **Activity 4.5**

1   Using the results from Activity 4.4, calculate and explain the ICER:

$$ICER = \frac{\text{Expected cost new chemotherapy} - \text{expected cost old chemotherapy}}{\text{Expected utility new chemotherapy} - \text{expected utility old chemotherapy}}$$

2   Compare the ICER with the average cost-effectiveness of each option and comment on the results.

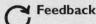 **Feedback**

1   $ICER = \dfrac{341.47 - 235.30}{0.97 - 0.96} = \dfrac{106.17}{0.01} = £10,671$ per QALY gained (but note, if you had calculated this using DATA Tree Age without rounding, the answer would have been £13.78, which shows the impact of rounding errors!).

2   The average cost-effectiveness ratios for the old and new chemotherapies are 245 and 353 respectively. The estimates give much lower figures but are not the right figures for comparison because they don't give the true picture of the additional cost of benefits gained over and above existing treatment. The ICER value of £13,782 is the cost of the additional gain per additional QALY.

Testing results using sensitivity analysis

The results provided in Activity 4.5 represent the 'base case' scenario where the best estimates are used. However, in populating a decision tree with probabilities and values you may find that data are not available or its value disputed. In such cases, the impact of changing the variable should be examined (something you will learn about in Chapters 14 and 15).

 Activity 4.6

Reviewing the feedback to Activity 4.4:

1 Consider how you might test the reliability (robustness) of the model.
2 Consider the advantages and disadvantages of using this model to make a decision on whether to replace the old with the new chemotherapy.

 Feedback

1 All inputs to the model can be changed. However, in this particular example, the variables most likely to affect the results are:

- *probability of hospitalization*: because the cost is so much greater, a relatively small change in the probability is likely to affect the results
- *probability of having a side-effect* because this is the main influence on the proportion of costs incurred
- *price of the drug* because it is a policy variable

2 The *advantages* are that the model forces a systematic decision to be made with all values explicit and easily examined, and no data processing errors. This particular model is also simple and easy to communicate. If the sensitivity analysis showed that results were very sensitive to a less reliable variable, it could also indicate where further research was needed to clarify this variable (such as the probability of side-effects). The *disadvantages* are that time still has to be taken to communicate and explain the nature of the decision to policy-makers. It is also possible that the model may be considered too simplistic and questions may be raised about: a) the possibility of patients needing ambulatory and hospital care; b) a longer-term impact of chemotherapy drugs; and c) the possibility of side-effects recurring in the future – neither of the latter two problems can be accounted for with a decision tree model.

Summary

You have learnt about the use of modelling in decision-making and worked through the design of a decision tree. This illustrated how to: define problems; set up model structures; assign and apply probabilities; assign values to consequences; calculate expected values of each option; and interpret the results. You will now learn about another approach, Markov modelling.

References

Claxton K and Posnett J (1996) An economic approach to clinical trial design and research priority-setting. *Health Economics* 5(6): 513–24.
Nuitjen MJC (1999) The selection of data sources for use in modelling studies, in G Malarky (ed.) *Economic evaluation in healthcare*. Auckland: Adis Books, pp. 117–29.

Further reading

Goldie SJ and Corso PS (2003) Decision analysis, in AC Haddix, SM Teutch, PA Shaffer and D Dunet (eds) *Prevention effectiveness: A guide to decision analysis and economic evaluation.* Oxford: Oxford University Press, pp. 103–26.

Muennig P (2002) Constructing a model, in *Designing and conducting cost-effectiveness analysis in medicine and health care.* San Francisco: Jossey-Bass, pp. 167–89.

In 1997 in the *Journal of American Medical Association* a series of five papers 'primers on medical decision analysis' were written by a combined team of Detsky, Naglie, Krahn, Redelmeier and Naimark and serve as a good introduction to the topic. Several of the papers are available on the internet.

5 | Introduction to Markov modelling

Overview

In this chapter you will be introduced to the reasons for using Markov modelling and learn about the structure of a basic Markov model. You will see how a model might be constructed and developed further in practice and the limitations of such modelling. The chapter ends by presenting a framework to help judge the quality of modelling papers.

Learning objectives

After working through this chapter, you will be able to:

- **explain under what circumstances Markov models are used in economic evaluation**
- **describe how Markov models work and how they are used to estimate effectiveness, costs and cost-effectiveness**
- **interpret the results of Markov models and critically appraise the underlying assumptions**

Key terms

Markov cycle The equal periods of time that the overall time horizon of a model is divided into and during which all information about people is held constant.

Markov state Markov models assume that at any stage in a Markov process a patient should always be in one of a finite number of defined health states.

Probabilistic Any event is based on chance, randomness or probability – it can't be predicted exactly but the likelihood of the event occurring is known.

Probabilistic sensitivity analysis A method of analysis that explicitly incorporates parameter uncertainty. The defining point is that variables are specified as distributions rather than point estimates as in a deterministic analysis.

Transition matrix Summary of the transition probabilities between all Markov states in a model.

Transition probability The probability of moving from one Markov state to another at the end of a Markov cycle.

Uncertainty Where the true value of a parameter or the true structure of a process is unknown.

Introduction

There are two key limitations with decision trees. First, their structure only allows progress of a patient through the model in one way (as they are read, from left to right) and so people are not allowed to move back and forth between states. Therefore, decision trees may not be very suitable for some health conditions where there are recurrent events (such as chronic diseases). Second, a decision tree does not have a temporal element, in other words all events happen at a single time point. Therefore, if anything happens at other periods of time or sequentially it has to be calculated outside the model and entered in at the terminal node stage.

Markov models (named after the Russian mathematician Andrey Andreyevich Markov) are able to handle both of these issues with ease and are therefore better at representing more complex processes happening over time. They can also reduce the size of decision trees and present options more clearly, both of which can reduce the number of errors made as well as ease presentation of the ideas represented in a model.

Markov models are concerned with the condition of a (group of) patient(s) varying over time and can represent a series of events that unfold over time. They are particularly appropriate for recurring processes and for care of patients with chronic diseases.

What is a Markov model?

Markov models assume that there are finite numbers of defined health states (so-called Markov states) and at any time each patient should be assigned to one (and only one) health state. At the end of each cycle, there is a risk of a patient moving from one state of health to another, defined by transition probabilities. Transition probabilities can depend on the current time (e.g. the chance of death increases with time due to ageing, independent of health). The probabilities of moving from one state to all other possible states should always add up to 1.

Having identified a decision problem (as for decision trees and economic evaluations) and the health states, Figure 5.1 shows a decision tree with Markov nodes and rounded branches to the sub-tree indicating where the Markov process begins. The number and the definition of health states will depend on the nature of the policy question but as the number of health states increases the model gets more complex. The model in Figure 5.1 would enable you to determine the number of healthy people and the number of people who died at the end of each time interval (i.e. cycle); therefore, there are only two Markov states defined: healthy or dead.

There are seven steps in setting up a Markov model:

1 Identify the Markov states and the allowable transitions.
2 Choose the length of the cycle.
3 Find out and set the initial and transition probabilities.
4 Give values ('pay-offs') to the outcomes in the model.
5 Set the 'stopping' rule.
6 Decide on the process for analysis.
7 Test the validity of the model.

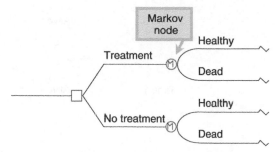

Figure 5.1 Decision tree for comparing treatment vs. no treatment

Identify the Markov states and the allowable transitions

The first steps to identify the Markov states related to the relevant clinical scenarios. States might include health, dead, disease stage, treatment status and/or other significant events that trigger an outcome or cost. Each state identified must be mutually exclusive, so a person cannot be in more than one state at any one time. They must also cover all relevant states exhaustively. The narrower the definition of 'states' the larger the number of states needed, the more complex a model becomes, and the quantity of data needed to populate the model increases. Therefore there should only be a finite, feasibly small, set of states defined.

Each state is represented by a circle or oval. Transitions between the states are shown with a series of arrows. The simplest type of Markov model is illustrated in Figure 5.2. This shows two states, alive and dead. This model allows transitions from alive to dead, whereas there is no exit from the Dead state, which is therefore an 'absorbing' state. The arrows from each circle back into themselves showing that some people will stay in that state from one time cycle to the next. It would be possible for arrows to go both to and from two states to illustrate the ability to move from one state to another.

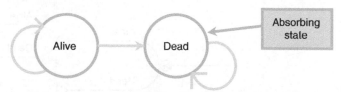

Figure 5.2 States and allowable transitions for a simple Markov model

Figure 5.2 can also be represented graphically as a series of states over time. Figure 5.3 shows the movement over time periods for the simple model where everyone begins by being alive.

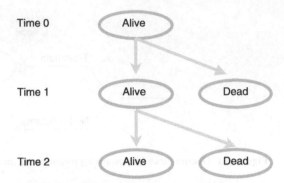

Figure 5.3 Graphical representation of simple Markov model over two time periods

✎ Activity 5.1

1 Draw the decision tree structure for a Markov model for Figure 5.2.
2 Imagine a Markov model with three states: healthy, ill and dead. Try to draw the states and possible transitions between the states using the same type of format as Figure 5.2. (Hint: note that some arrows will be missing or uni-directional. This task should become clearer when you encounter examples in this chapter. You should revisit this task if you do not fully understand it at this stage.)

↻ Feedback

1 It is possible that once people reach the terminal nodes they are shuttled back to the beginning of the Markov process, unless they reach an 'absorbing state'. This reflects the recursive nature of Markov models. A decision tree would need a very large number of sub-trees in order to capture this. There is another way of representing this Markov process, where M in the circle denotes it is a Markov chain (see Figure 5.4).

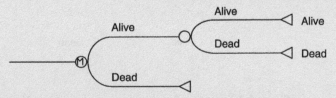

Figure 5.4 Decision tree structure for a Markov model

2 Figure 5.5 shows that from the state 'healthy' it is possible to remain healthy, die or become ill in the next period. From the state 'ill' people could become healthy, remain ill or die in the next period. This explains why there are bi-directional arrows between health and ill. Once a person is dead, they remain dead so there is only one circular arrow that goes out and back into the same state.

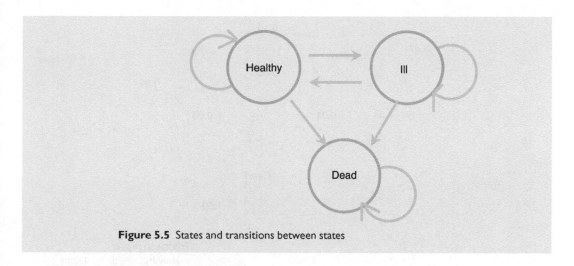

Figure 5.5 States and transitions between states

Choose the length of the cycle

The analytical horizon of a Markov model is divided into equal increments of time (the 'Markov cycle') that represent the minimum amount of time any one person will spend in a state before transition to another state is possible. Throughout the duration of any cycle, all information about subjects is held constant. At the end of the cycle the model re-evaluates the position of everyone to decide what proportion of the population moves from one state to another and what proportion remains in the same state. All these transitions are defined in terms of probabilities.

The length of the Markov cycle should be no shorter than the minimum amount of time required for moving from one state to another. This might reflect the biological processes of the specific disease modelled and/or the frequency of specific economic events including treatment. However, in practice the cycle length may also be determined by the availability of data. The length of cycle you set may be short (one hour) or long (e.g. years). Shorter cycles can be more burdensome in terms of computer time depending on the total time period covered by the analysis.

Find out and set the initial and transition probabilities

In a Markov model, each move from one state to another is determined by the transition probabilities. The sum of transition probabilities from each state must equal 1.0. Figure 5.6 adds transition probabilities to the model from Activity 5.1 and shows the accompanying transition matrix. Assuming a Markov cycle of one year, this would mean that of those who are ill, 92% of patients remain ill one year later, 3% would be dead one year later and 5% would recover.

Furthermore, the initial distribution of the cohort across different Markov states can be defined. For example, at the beginning of the Markov process you can assume that everyone is alive but 20% of the cohort had already contracted the disease. In this case, the initial probabilities of starting the process as a healthy

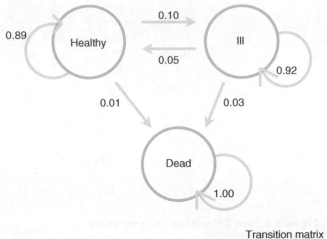

Transition matrix

	Healthy	Ill	Dead
Healthy	0.89	0.10	0.01
Ill	0.05	0.92	0.03
Dead	0	0	1.0

Figure 5.6 Markov model with transition probabilities

person are 0.80, ill 0.20 and dead 0.0. In other words, if you are following 100 people, 80 people will start in healthy state, 20 people will be ill and no one will be dead. Note that the initial probabilities are completely different from transition probabilities and are only used to define the initial distribution of people in each state before you start running the model.

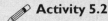 **Activity 5.2**

The transition matrix (Table 5.1) adds in another state for ill health.

1 Calculate the missing probabilities in Table 5.1.
2 Draw the revised model in the style of Figure 5.6 to include the new state.

Table 5.1 Transition matrix

	Healthy	Ill	Severely ill	Dead
Healthy	0.89	0.06	?	0.01
Ill	0.05	?	0.18	0.02
Severely ill	0	0.19	0.73	?
Dead	0	0	?	1.0

Feedback

1 Remember that the transitional probabilities of moving from one state to all other possible states should always add up to 1. Therefore, the missing probabilities, by row, are: healthy (0.04), ill (0.75), severely ill (0.08), dead (0).

2 See Figure 5.7.

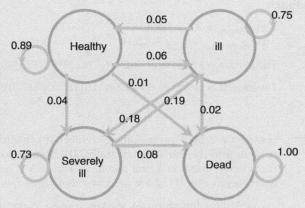

Figure 5.7 Revised Markov model including the new state, severely ill

As with decision models, there are a variety of sources of data to estimate transition probabilities, as you will see in Chapter 6. However, it is likely that some data in the literature will need to be converted as most of the relevant information available is given as a rate (number of events from 0 to infinity that occur over a set unit of time, e.g. four people with severe pneumonia in a population of 298 hospital admissions for pneumonia) not as a probability (a number between 0 and 1). Alternatively, data can be reported over a different time period to the cycles represented in a model (e.g. reporting the number of events from a cohort over five years, when a model cycle is only one year).

Activity 5.3

Assume you have selected a *one year cycle* for your Markov model. You have the following information that you want to convert into two different probabilities for your Markov model:

a) 33 people per year in a population of 100 have a side-effect in one year
b) every three months 23 people from the sample of 500 experience an asthma attack.

Use the formula below to convert each rate into a probability (*p*)

$$p = 1 - e^{-rt}$$

Where: e = base of natural logarithm (equals to 2.7182818 . . .); r = rate; t = time period.

You will need to substitute values into the equation and consider the time period you are asked for and information given.

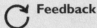 **Feedback**

   a) $p_{\text{side-effect}} = 1 - 2.7182818^{-(0.33*(12/12))} = 0.28$
   b) $p_{\text{asthma attack}} = 1 - 2.7182818^{-((23/500)*((12/3)))} = 0.168$

The formula in EXCEL is $=(1-(EXP(-1*(0.33*(12/12)))))$

The formula in EXCEL is $=(1-(EXP(-1*((23/500)*(12/3)))))$

Setting the initial probabilities involves organizing the hypothetical group of patients into the initial health states. The appropriate distribution will depend on the specific question being asked. In Figure 5.1, for example, 100% of patients would begin alive if the question was about life expectancy from birth.

An important limitation of Markov models is the inherent assumption that the current state of health of a patient is sufficient to predict the next state. This means that even if one person experiences a particular health state more often, in the process of working through the model, they are no more or less likely than another person to have another recurrence in the future. However, in real life the probabilities of moving to a particular health state may be increased or decreased depending on the previous experiences of the patient. For example, the risk of having venous thrombus is much greater if the patient had a previous thromboembolic event. This 'memoryless' feature of Markov models can be worked around by creating health states dependent on history or by adding additional health states, but this is beyond the scope of this introduction.

Give values to the outcomes in the model

Because Markov models run through cycles, outcomes such as costs or life years are accumulated all the way through the model rather than only at the end (as with decision trees). The simplest weighting would be to assume a weight of 1.0 for being alive and 0.0 for being dead. If this was done for Figure 5.2 and the model run over many annual cycles, summing the weights at each cycle (year) and dividing by the size of the cohort would give the average life expectancy in years, as each completed cycle would be counted as 1. Attaching weights between 0 and 1 to states for each annual cycle to reflect quality of life would allow calculation of QALYs.

As costs are also represented as outcomes in such models, weights for costs are attached in the same way as outcomes. Therefore the probability of a cost occurring is multiplied by the cost of an event within a cycle and summed over each cycle to present total costs over time. One of the advantages of Markov models is that these costs (or outcomes), which may occur at different time periods, can be easily discounted within this framework using the standard discounting formula for net present value (NPV):

$$NPV = V_t / (1+r)^t, \text{ where } V_t = \text{value at time t and } r = \text{discount rate}$$

The NPVs from each intervention are added up to calculate the ICER. Further details on discounting are given in Chapter 12.

Activity 5.4

1 Using the transition matrix from Figure 5.6 and assuming that a cohort of 1000 people begin the process alive and that cycles last for one year each:

a) calculate how many people will be healthy, ill and dead at the end of the third cycle
b) consider how you would change the probabilities of death in the model
c) calculate life expectancy at the beginning of the four year follow-up stage for the healthy state, ill state and overall.

2 Assuming the outcome weight is changed to 0.5 for those in the ill state, calculate the number of QALYs accumulated for the cohort at the end of the third cycle.
3 If outcomes were discounted at a rate of 3%, what would be the total number of QALYs at the end of each cycle (up to time 3)?

Feedback

1 a) The initial state is already defined, where everyone is healthy. So there are 1000 people in healthy state, and 0 for both ill and dead. When calculating the numbers for each cell, first think of the allowed transitions. For example, in this case only healthy people or ill people can transit to a healthy state from a previous cycle, whereas people from each stage can die (and all dead remain dead). For time 1, the probability of remaining healthy (if initially in healthy state) and the probability of getting healthy from ill state should be multiplied with the number of people in those states ($1000 \times 0.89 + 0 \times 0.05 = 890$). The rest of the calculations should follow the same rules. Note also that for each cycle (i.e. each row in the table) there should be a total of 1000 people (see Table 5.2).

Table 5.2 Calculation of numbers in each state

	Healthy	Ill	Dead
Time 0	1000	0	0
Time 1	890	100	10
Time 2	797	181	22
Time 3	719	246	35

b) The model assumes death has a constant probability over time of 0.01. Since the probability of death increases in an individual over time (after the age of 1 year), one possibility would be to define the probability of death as a mathematical function and amend the other probabilities accordingly to ensure they sum to 1.

c) If all live states are weighted as 1, the life expectancy can be calculated using the sum of weights in the columns healthy and ill divided by the size of the cohort (i.e. 3933/1000). Therefore the average life expectancy is 3.9 years at four-year follow-up. In the healthy state it is 3.4 years and in the ill state it is 0.5.

2 As you can see in Table 5.3 the total is 3406 + 263.5 = 3669.5 QALYs.

Table 5.3 Calculation of numbers in each state if outcome weight is 0.5

	Healthy	Ill	Dead
Time 0	1000	0	0
Time 1	890	50	10
Time 2	797	90.5	22
Time 3	719	123	35
Sum	3406	263.5	35

3 The 'reward' at the end of each cycle in terms of discounted QALYs is shown in Table 5.4.

Table 5.4 'Reward' at end of each cycle in terms of discounted QALYs

	Healthy	Ill	Dead
Time 0	0	0	0
Time 1	864	49	0
Time 2	751	85	0
Time 3	658	113	0

Set the 'stopping' rule

Eventually population cohorts die out over time. However, because the models are probabilistic the number of people declines exponentially but never quite reaches zero. Therefore a 'stopping rule' needs to be introduced to complete the Markov process. For example, approximate the time when all members of the population are dead (e.g. when 99.9% are dead). However, for many disease scenarios running the model for a limited time period (let's say for 20 years) would be sufficient, as beyond this time the policy question may become irrelevant due to unforeseeable developments (such as new treatment algorithms).

The stopping rule is used at the end of each cycle to determine whether the process should continue calculating. There are some software packages available for developing Markov models that predefine some stopping rules. For example, for DATA TREEAGE software, the automatic stopping rule is defined as '*stage >10&(_stage>100/_stage_reward<0.001)*'. This means that the process should not terminate before ten cycles are completed but before either a maximum 101 stages are complete or when the net reward (e.g. life years or QALYs) drops below a threshold of 0.001. All these conditions can be changed to reflect the nature of the problem being evaluated.

Decide on the process for analysis

The standard way to analyse a Markov model, and the approach used in this chapter to date, is using a 'cohort simulation' model where one group of people enter at the start and then move through the model (with no other groups of people following them into the model in the next time period). At the end of all transitions within the model, the percentage of people in each state is calculated. For example, running the model presented in Figure 5.6 for all stages of the model generates probabilities of being in each Markov state as shown in Figure 5.8 or alternatively proportions of the cohort in each state over time in Figure 5.9. Comparing such

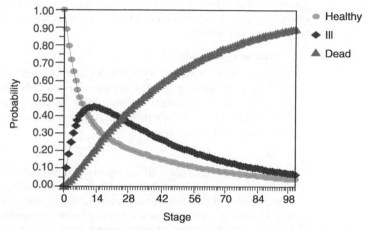

Figure 5.8 Markov probability analysis

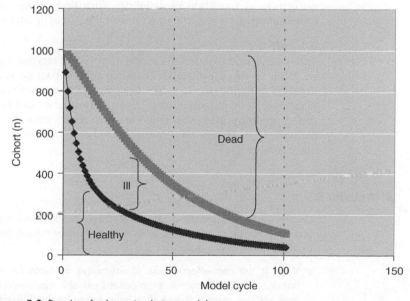

Figure 5.9 Results of cohort simulation model

profiles with and without treatment would provide evidence of the incremental impact of treatment. For example, if the intervention decreases the fatality from the disease by half (i.e. the transitional probability from ill to dead reduces from 0.03 to 0.015), then two identical cohorts are simulated using the different probabilities (one with and one without the treatment) and the cumulated results are compared.

Test the validity of the model

No fixed universal framework for evaluating the validity of models exists and, given the diversity of needs from modelling it is unlikely that one can be developed. However, Sculpher *et al.* (2000) do offer a broad framework to help examine three aspects of quality:

a. Structure of the model

Is the structure consistent with the decision problem and underlying theory of the disease? All assumptions of the model need to be specified, justified and the impact of relaxing assumptions examined. Specific parts of the model requiring closer examination include the options being compared, the disease states, time horizon and length of cycles.

b. Data

You need to present data in an open and accountable way and use the 'best available' data (which will be a function of time and budget available in relation to the impact of the variable on results). You should not use data selectively and should look first for evidence from systematic reviews/meta-analyses. Any data based on expert opinion should explain how experts were defined and sampled. Checks on how data have been incorporated into the model should be made e.g. calculation of transition probabilities, inclusion of half cycle correction and examination of 1st and 2nd order uncertainty (see Chapter 15).

c. Consistency

This is a check on whether the model does what it sets out to do. Internal consistency can be checked through examining the impact on results from changing variables to their extreme values or using a different software package with the same model to compare results. External consistency can be examined by comparing results at different time points with results from the literature (e.g. comparing 5, 10 or 15 year rates survival rates) or from similar models developed by other analysts.

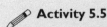 **Activity 5.5**

1 List the advantages and disadvantages of Markov models outlined in this chapter.
2 State which type of model (decision tree or Markov model) you would select to examine the following questions:

a) What is the cost-effectiveness of alternative methods for controlling Chagas disease? (Chagas disease is an infectious parasitic disease found mainly in Latin America. It is mostly caught after being bitten by the 'kissing bug'. In the initial acute phase of illness symptoms are usually mild and can include fever, headache, anorexia, conjunctivitis and mycocarditis for two to three months after which the disease goes into remission for many years. In the longer-term chronic phase cardiomyopathy and congestive health failure may develop followed by death from heart disease.)

b) What is the cost-effectiveness of alternative approaches to antenatal screening for Down's syndrome? (Down's syndrome is a congenital disorder, caused by the presence of an extra 21st chromosome, in which the affected person has mild to moderate mental retardation, short stature and a flattened facial profile.)

c) Should the number of routine episiotomies be reduced from 60% to 30%? (episiotomy is surgically cutting to widen the vaginal opening for birth).

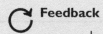 **Feedback**

1

Advantages	Disadvantages
• Models events as they change over time • Models movements in chronic disease in a person's life and therefore is better able to reflect the complexity of disease • Captures the impact of time within models • Can predict value of policies at different time points • Can handle costs and effects simultaneously and assess covariance of these variables (in simulation models) • With more advanced modelling skills, many of the disadvantages can be accounted for • Discounting can be applied easily	• Occurrence of an event is not dependent on history of events (model has no memory) • Computing time needed (especially for individual simulation models) • Requires specific computing packages • Level of knowledge required to specify the structure of the model and functional forms for relationships within model • More complex models may compromise the transparency

2 a) Markov model: the impact of Chagas disease is long term and whilst some acute events may occur within a few years, the main health impact occurs over 25 years later and can last for 10 years or more.

b) Decision tree: the decision will focus on the number of cases identified, which will occur in less than nine months.

c) Decision tree: the choice of treatment and impact from episiotomy is experienced in the short term. Outcomes could be vaginal tearing or need for suturing and the intervention is unlikely to have much impact on the health of the baby.

Summary

You have learnt about the reasons for using Markov modelling and the seven steps in setting up a model: identifying the states and allowable transitions; choosing the length of the cycle; finding out and setting the initial and transition probabilities; giving values to the outcomes; setting the 'stopping' rule; deciding on the process for the analysis; and testing the validity of the model. Having completed the first section of the book on the structure of economic evaluation, you will now learn about how resources used in health care can be measured and valued.

References

Sculpher M, Fenwick E, Claxton K (2000) Assessing quality in decision analytic cost-effectiveness models: a suggested framework and example of application. *Pharmacoeconomics* 17: 461–77.

Further reading

Decision tree and Markov models can be developed using MS Excel software. However, to work through models in practice, you may wish to try to access some decision analysis software, as this may be more user-friendly and fit for purpose. Occasionally it is possible to use a package as a free trial for a limited period.

DATA TREEAGE (http://treeage.com). This is an easy to use package that encompasses both decision trees and Markov modelling. It has a helpful analytical approach to qualitative and probabilistic sensitivity analysis and the manual provides clear tutorial guidance for using the package. It is for Windows-based computers only.

Decision Makers (http://nemc.org/medicine/cdm/dmaker1.htm). This is a powerful package and able to conduct Markov analyses. It requires a DOS system to run for any IBM-compatible computer.

Precision Tree (http://palisade.com) and @Risk. These are add-on packages for use in Excel and can be used for decision trees and Markov models with a range of sensitivity analyses fully supported within the programme.

Reuter M, Hennig J, Netter P, Buehner M and Hueppe M (2004) Using latent mixed Markov models for the choice of the best pharmacological treatment. *Statistics in Medicine* 23(9):1337–49.

SECTION 2

Measuring and valuing resource use

6 | Cost of health services

Overview

This chapter focuses on the resources used and saved by health care providers as a result of adopting a particular course of action. There are three stages when assessing the costs of health services: identification, measurement and valuation. It is generally useful to maintain a distinction between the quantification of resource use in physical terms and the valuation of resource use in money terms when reporting results. The perspective adopted in economic evaluation is one of identifying opportunity costs.

Learning objectives

After working through this chapter, you will be able to:

- **explain which changes in resource use to include in any economic evaluation**
- **describe the different methods which can be used to measure changes in resource use**
- **describe some of the main sources of secondary data on health service costs**

Key terms

Purchasing power parities Rates of currency conversion that equalize the purchasing power of different currencies.

Introduction

Resources are severely limited in the health sector, especially in low-income countries, and policy-makers must make choices between different health care interventions and strategies to meet health targets. Cost is one of the many factors which should be taken into account when choosing.

Resource use is measured not in monetary form but in natural or physical units. For example, different types of resources used in health care are staff, equipment, materials and drugs. Often resource use is measured in terms of aggregates such as outpatient visits, inpatient days or admissions, operations and laboratory tests, rather than the individual inputs, such as staff time, combined to produce an inpatient day. These quantities are then valued in monetary terms by multiplying by the appropriate unit cost or input price. There are some inputs where it may be simpler to proceed directly to monetary valuation, for example, out-of-pocket expenses incurred by patients in seeking and obtaining treatment.

Which resources to include?

Which resources to include depends primarily on the perspective of the analysis. If a societal perspective is adopted all resources used to provide interventions and all future resources 'saved' by the success of the intervention should be included. When a narrower perspective is adopted, such as that of the health care sector or of a particular organization, changes in resource use elsewhere in the economy or outside of the organization are ignored. The focus is firmly on resource costs. Generally, when assessing cost-effectiveness, instances where there is no change in resource use are not relevant. The main category of events is transfer payments where one group are better off and another are worse off but no resources are consumed. For example, if an individual is returned to health and consequently resumes paid employment the other taxpayers gain in that this individual will now make greater tax payments and also payments (from tax revenue) to the individual will reduce.

One of the unresolved methodological questions with respect to measuring and valuing the change in resource use as a result of a particular intervention concerns future health service costs. These can be classified as:

- related, occurring in years of life lived anyway;
- unrelated, occurring in years of life lived anyway;
- related, occurring in years of life gained; and
- unrelated, occurring in years of life gained.

The most contentious of these are unrelated costs arising in the years of life gained. One suggestion is that the measurement of costs be guided by the measurement of effectiveness. Only if effectiveness is measured with respect to total mortality (rather than condition-specific mortality) should unrelated health service costs be included. Quite reasonably, if all the future QALYs that are anticipated for this group of patients are to be included, all the future costs required in order to provide these QALYs should be included. Whatever policy is adopted there will be practical challenges. On the one hand, if unrelated costs are to be included, they can be difficult to forecast accurately. On the other hand, if the decision is to exclude these costs, it will sometimes be difficult to distinguish related from unrelated costs.

How to measure resource use?

There are a number of potential sources of data on resource use including randomized trials, administrative databases, clinical databases and medical records. A summary description and outline of their advantages and disadvantages are presented in Table 6.1. The issue of how to measure resource use has often been seen in terms of economic analysis alongside randomized trials versus economic modelling which combines data from a potentially wide range of sources. This is a false

Table 6.1 Comparison of data sources

Data source	Description	Advantages	Disadvantages
Clinical trials	A planned therapeutic, diagnostic or preventive study involving people and comparing concurrently one intervention with another or with a placebo or with no intervention to determine their relative safety and efficacy in a controlled environment	Careful design means that internal validity is high as impact of confounding variables is minimized	Because of strict inclusion and exclusion criteria results often have little external validity (i.e. results are not easily transferable to populations outside a trial setting)
Meta-analyses	Statistical technique for summarizing results of multiple quantitative studies. Involves computing an effect size for the same variable in each study and calculating a mean effect	Greater statistical power than individual studies to detect small but consistent effects. Can be used when comparator in economic analysis is not the same as the comparator in a clinical trial or when clinical trials have only one arm. Useful for estimates of treatment failure	May be subject to inclusion and publication bias. It is of questionable validity when there are small numbers of trials and when studies are heterogeneous. Same problems with external validity as individual trials
Administrative databases	Database recording all use of health care made by individuals	Large numbers of patients and high external validity. Good for probabilities of health service utilization across levels of service	Little on clinical outcomes. Often little detail from hospitalizations. Patients are not randomized and no control groups possible. Population may not be representative of general population
Clinical databases	Specialized databases of patients with a specific condition or using specific interventions	May have long-term follow-up data and collect data on a wider range of clinical outcomes, including detailed information on the health of patients	Incomplete information on health care use. External validity may be compromised depending on person/site(s) collecting data. Patients not randomized

Table 6.1 *Continued*

Data source	Description	Advantages	Disadvantages
Medical records	Records held by clinicians on condition and care of individual patients. May be held separately by institution or as linked information across institutions	Records actual rather than assumed care. Can link outcomes to diagnosis	Different types of records held by inpatients and outpatients. Data search and entry can be time-consuming. Access may be complicated by privacy protection. Data is often illegible and partial
Consensus development techniques	Approaches used to obtain expert opinion and consensus of this opinion	Useful where there is no or little published evidence or where evidence is conflicting, unreliable or insufficient	Methods are used with variable stringency. No guidance on who is included as an expert and each brings uncontrollable biases. Impact of outliers from a small group of experts is large. If used iteratively, dropout can be a problem

Source: Adapted from Nuitjen (1999)

dichotomy in that economic analysis alongside randomized trials will almost invariably involve elements of modelling and economic modelling will generally utilize data from trials (should suitable data be available).

However, economic evaluation is increasingly turning to economic modelling rather than economic analysis alongside trials. There are two main advantages: first, the evaluation can be designed to address the question facing decision-makers (in contrast, trials often do not address precisely the choices faced by decision-makers); second, economic models can utilize information from a wide range of sources as opposed to a single study. The analysis is then not subject to the data limitations of any one particular study. This second advantage is clearly not without its dangers and analysts have to be very careful with respect to the selection of which data to combine. The scope for manipulation of the eventual outcome in terms of cost-effectiveness is probably greater in a model than it is with economic analysis alongside a trial.

Randomized trials do have a number of advantages for estimating resource use. The quality of data is generally high. A trial involves prospective data collection. Also, the general standard of record-keeping is often higher than that in routine practice. It is possible to link the measurement of resource use with the measurement of clinical outcome. Randomization ensures that differences in resource use are more readily attributable to differences in the intervention and in response to the intervention as opposed to differences between patients. Individual patient data are more likely to be available which then permits more extensive statistical analysis.

However, there are several potential disadvantages as well. These stem largely from a single source – trials are rarely designed to evaluate cost-effectiveness. They are primarily concerned with safety and effectiveness. In order to achieve high internal validity the patients and centres selected may be unrepresentative of those encountered in routine practice. Many trials are of too short a duration to capture all of the resource consequences of the intervention. The sample size is determined with respect to the primary clinical outcome and may not be large enough to reflect adequately the resource implications. For example, there may be a small number of patients with particularly high costs and if the sample is too small they may be over- or more likely under-represented. The collection of cost data is often not given as high a priority as the collection of clinical data.

Another concern is that some costs might arise in trials but not in routine clinical practice. At first sight it seems clear that costs associated with conducting the trial should be omitted and this is in general the accepted position. However, separation of trial costs from service costs will not always be easy and also it is possible that part of any change in outcome which is achieved is as a result of resources consumed as a result of the conduct of the trial. The extent to which this is a problem will depend largely on the extent to which the trial does or doesn't closely reflect routine practice.

Whatever the source of data on resource use, a general lack of good quality data is a feature of most studies. Studies are always constrained with respect to the resources available to collect data and difficult judgements must be made about where to invest these scarce resources.

 Activity 6.1

Suppose that you have been asked to undertake an economic evaluation of a cardio-vascular screening and intervention programme led by community nurses. The aim of the programme is to reduce blood pressure, blood cholesterol level, and smoking and thus reduce subsequent heart disease and stroke. Suppose a randomized trial of the intervention is about to start.

1 Identify the range of different costs which you might wish to include in your analysis, assuming you are adopting a health service perspective.
2 Indicate which of these you would be able to get data on from the trial and which would require you to look elsewhere.

 Feedback

1 Taking a health service perspective, you might have suggested:

Direct costs of the whole intervention

- programme costs (e.g. nurse time, consumables, building costs)
- drug costs

- broader health service costs (doctor time)
- hospitalizations due to heart disease

General illness costs

- costs of treating other illnesses arising from the intervention (e.g. where a visit to a nurse identified other illnesses which required treatment)
- costs of treating other illnesses unrelated to the intervention (e.g. inpatient costs for an unrelated accident)

Future costs

- related costs arising in years of life lived anyway (e.g. the costs associated with treatment of stroke, if these are affected by the intervention)
- related costs arising in years of life gained (e.g. the costs of treating all coronary events in the life years gained)

Trial costs

- costs of the research team and costs of any tests undertaken only for the purposes of the research

2 Data on the direct costs of the intervention could be collected in the trial, as could trial costs. Some of the information on general illness costs could come from the trial but not all of it. It is unlikely that data on future costs will be available from the trial.

 Activity 6.2

What are the main advantages and disadvantages of estimating costs by collecting information alongside a randomized trial?

 Feedback

The advantages are the high accuracy of the data and the likelihood that differences in cost do reflect treatment differences. The potential disadvantages are that the costs observed in a trial may not be a good guide to costs in routine clinical practice and that the period of follow-up and the sample size may be inadequate.

Valuing resources

The two key principles underlying the valuation of resource use are opportunity cost and marginal cost. The opportunity cost of resources is not necessarily what was paid for them but rather their value in their best alternative use. In certain circumstances the operation of markets will establish prices which are equal to these opportunity costs and where possible you can use market prices because they are the best guide as to the value of the resources. However, market prices might be distorted owing to taxes or subsidies, in which case the price is a less accurate measure of the marginal value of a unit of the resource. A specific problem can arise with respect to one particular price, namely the exchange rate. When comparing costs from different countries it is tempting to use the exchange rate between the two currencies to convert the costs from one currency to the other. However, official exchange rates are not always a good guide to the value of one currency in terms of another. The comparison of spending in different countries using exchange rates is potentially misleading because it fails to take account of differences in price levels. Purchasing power parity is used as an alternative to exchange rates in order to facilitate comparisons in spending between countries. It is the rate of currency conversion at which a given amount of currency will purchase the same volume of goods and services in two countries. This topic is explored more fully in Chapter 18 which examines the transferability of results.

Not all inputs are traded in markets and in such circumstances alternative procedures are required. The next chapter examines the example of the time given by informal carers.

Because of the incremental nature of economic evaluation, you will generally be interested in marginal costs rather than average costs. Marginal cost is the change in total cost when producing an additional unit of output. The marginal cost of an activity depends on the time frame of the analysis. As an approximation it is quite common to estimate marginal cost using average costs. This is done because average cost is generally easier to measure. In the long run, average costs will be a good approximation to marginal costs since all inputs, including labour and capital, become variable, but generally speaking average costs are not a good approximation in the short run where many costs may be fixed and only a few may be variable. For example, staff time (and its associated cost) may be fixed in the short run, whereas drug costs will generally be variable. One specific instance of the variability of marginal cost arises where over a certain range of output additional units are readily produced without many additional resources, whereas when full capacity is reached the production of additional units may require many more additional resources.

Data collection techniques

Assuming that a study is going to collect some primary data rather than rely wholly on secondary sources, there are a variety of methods by which these data can be collected. Forms are commonly used to extract information on the use of hospital services. Medical records can be an invaluable source of data. However, there are frequently problems with missing data and also the information is specific to health services. Where adequate records are unavailable, questionnaires given to patients or to their carers can be a means of documenting past resource use. They are of course dependent on patient recall which may well be biased and also, in the absence of good response rates, may be unrepresentative. Patient diaries can be a good way of identifying resource use outside of hospitals where detailed records may not be kept or may be widely dispersed making data collection costly. However, such enrolling of patients in the data collection exercise needs a high level of compliance if the data are to be representative and also diaries will work best when the patient has regular contact with members of the research team and if the data collection period is not too long.

Clinical databases of patients with specific conditions or patients undergoing a particular intervention are another valuable means of capturing data on longer-term resource use. They can supplement information collected in trials, which frequently have too short a period in which patients are followed up. Also, clinical databases generally cover many more patients than trials and thus are better able to capture important but relatively uncommon resource-using events.

Sources of price/cost data for resource use in the health sector

The most ambitious international dataset on costs and input prices (WHO-CHOICE) has been assembled by the Global Programme on Evidence for Health Policy of the WHO (Adam *et al.* 2003; Johns *et al.* 2003). This work started in 1998 with the development of standard tools and methods and represents the first systematic attempt to estimate unit costs at both the patient and programme level for health care interventions in all countries and regions of the world. This facilitates the generation of unit costs that are not only consistent across interventions within one country but also allows for comparison across countries with similar determinants such as incidence and prevalence of diseases and socioeconomic factors. It also allows the estimation of the cost of scaling up interventions to different coverage levels by varying capacity utilization.

In addition to such cross-country datasets, there also exist numerous national datasets of unit costs within high-income countries. The most comprehensive cost data come from the United States where efficiency concerns within the publicly financed Medicare programme for the elderly led to new methods for measuring costs on a diagnosis basis. Sources of cost data in the US include: hospital charges adjusted using cost to charge ratios; data from internal hospital costing systems; diagnosis-related group payments for hospitalizations; and resource-based relative value units for physician services. In the UK a national reference costs dataset is produced by the Department of Health (2002), the main purpose of which is to provide a basis for comparison within (and outside) the NHS, at the level of individual treatments. A comprehensive dataset on health and social care costs in the UK is produced by Curtis and Netten (2004) and updated annually. Data on hospital costs are readily available for a number of other countries including France, Germany and Italy.

Datasets of costs in low-income countries are harder to find and there is a heavier reliance on specific costing studies for particular diseases or hospitals (Mulligan *et al.* 2003). There are studies using generally available hospital information reported to government. The major limitation of such studies is that while recording how much has been spent and on what, they do not enable the identification of the cost of providing specific health services. Many studies are now available which record the actual costs of providing health services in low-income countries. However, comparisons between studies must be made with care because different studies often use different costing methodologies. Also, the cost estimates are usually relevant to a specific setting and thus cannot be assumed to be representative of costs across a range of settings in that country.

Activity 6.3

> The mean cost of primary hip replacement in the UK in 2002 was £4356 and the range was from £2076 to £8150. What factors might explain this range of estimated costs?

 Feedback

> There will be marked differences with respect to the number of replacements undertaken in different centres and this will influence the costs. There will be differences in case mix: for example, some centres may have older and frailer patients necessitating longer lengths of stay. Different centres may use different replacement joints (at different prices). There may also be some differences with respect to the cost of inputs because of market forces. Finally, while all hospitals will have received the same guidance on costing methods there may be some differences in how these have been applied.

Summary

You have learned how to identify which resources to include when costing an intervention and its impact, distinguishing related and unrelated future health care use. You went on to learn about how to measure resource use including the merits and limitations of different data sources. Finally you considered how resources can be valued and data collected.

References

Adam T, Evans D and Murray C (2003) Econometric estimation of country-specific hospital costs. *Cost-Effectiveness and Resource Allocation* 1(3): 3, www.resource-allocation.com.

Curtis L and Netten A (2004) *Unit costs of health and social care 2004*. Canterbury: Personal Social Services Research Unit, University of Kent, www.pssru.ac.uk/uc/uc2004.htm.

Department of Health (2002) *NHS Reference Costs 2002*. London: Department of Health, www.dh.gov.uk/.

Johns B, Baltussen R and Hutubessy R (2003) Programme costs in the economic evaluation of health interventions. *Cost-Effectiveness and Resource Allocation* 1(1): 1, www.resource-allocation.com.

Mulligan J, Fox-Rushby J, Adam T, Johns B and Mills A (2003) *Unit costs of health care inputs in low and middle income regions*, DCPP Working Paper No. 9, September 2003, (www.fic.nih.gov/dcpp/wps/wp9.pdf).

Nuitjen MJC (1999) The selection of data sources for use in modelling studies, in G. Malarky (ed.) *Economic evaluation in healthcare*. Auckland: Adis Books, pp. 117–29.

Further reading

International Comparison Programme 2003–2006 Handbook, www.worldbank.org.

Luce BR, Manning WG, Siegel JE and Lipscomb J (1996) Estimating costs in cost-effectiveness analysis, in MR Gold, JE Siegel, LB Russell and MC Weinstein (eds) *Cost-effectiveness in health and medicine*. New York: Oxford University Press.

7 Valuation of non-health service resources

Overview

Decisions over what health services to provide have cost implications not only for health services but also for patients and their families. There are potentially important consequences in terms of non-health service resources. Seeking and receiving health care takes up the time of patients and of other household members. Successful treatment will allow patients and other household members to use their time differently in the future. These activities may be market or non-market in nature.

Learning objectives

After working through this chapter, you will be able to:

- **describe the range of indirect costs which are potentially relevant for purposes of economic evaluation**
- **discuss the advantages and disadvantages of different methods of data collection**
- **explain the main methods used to value non-market activities**

Key terms

Human capital The characteristics of people that allow them to earn a wage.

Introduction

First you will be introduced to production gains and losses as a result of receiving treatment. Then you will learn about the measurement and valuation of changes in time devoted to non-market activities as a consequence of health care. The time in question may be either that of the patient or of household members or other unpaid carers. These consequences of seeking and receiving care are sometimes referred to as indirect costs to distinguish them from the direct costs of health care (the goods and services consumed in the provision of health care which you learnt about in the preceding chapter).

Production gains

The issue of what to include or exclude when taking into account the return of sick workers to employment has been a source of confusion for many, in particular once the role of government is included. Consequently a number of different approaches have been adopted. Dolan and Olsen (2002) provide a clear-sighted account that incidentally also provides a nice example of the issue of transfer payments (where one group gains and another loses but no resources are used up).

As summarized in Table 7.1, on return to work the worker gains their after tax wage (W–T) and loses their sickness benefit (SB). The employer pays a wage (W) and receives a production gain (PG), while government gains taxation (T) and saves on sickness benefits (SB). The net change is simply the production gain. Taxation and sickness benefits are simply transfer payments from one group to another – for each gain there is a matching loss. If the distribution of gainers and losers is a concern it would of course be relevant to record such changes but they do not affect the cost-effectiveness of the intervention as such, which is determined by the incremental change in resource use relative to the incremental change in health outcome.

Table 7.1 The return of a productive worker

	Worker	Employer	Government
Increased production		+PG	
Wage implications	+(W–T)	–W	+T
Sickness benefits	–SB		+SB

Note: W = wage, SB = sickness benefit, T = taxation, PG = production gain.
Source: Dolan and Olsen (2002)

The most common means of valuation is to adopt the human capital approach. What output is lost if an individual is unable to work? This output is generally estimated by using the individual's gross earnings. The underlying justification assumes that employers go on hiring labour until the value of the marginal contribution to output by an additional worker is just matched by the cost of employing them. (Strictly speaking this cost is not restricted to the wage paid but should also include any pension contributions made by the employer and any national insurance payments.) The main alternative approach to valuing production gains and losses is the friction cost method which explicitly recognizes that in many circumstance output is only lost temporarily, for example, where a replacement can be hired from a pool of unemployed workers. As a consequence this approach produces lower estimates of lost output. Although it appears conceptually superior it is used less often than the human capital approach because the data it requires are less readily available.

There still remains a question as to whether production gains should be taken into account. If assessments of cost-effectiveness were routinely to take into account such effects one implication would be that more productive groups would tend to be given priority over less productive groups. The treatment of diseases which have a more marked impact on those of working age would tend to receive more resources than diseases where the major impact is on the elderly. It has been argued that to the extent that these production gains result in increased private consumption rather than a contribution to the rest of society, they are of less significance.

Opportunity cost of time

Not everyone sells their labour in a market and even those who do spend only part of their time on such activities. How is time to be valued when the opportunity foregone is not paid employment? It is to these wider non-market activities you now turn.

In the UK and US over recent years there has been promotion of care in the community for groups such as the elderly, those with mental health problems and those with Alzheimer's disease. This involves the time of informal carers, friends, family, acquaintances or neighbours of a patient who provide care for which they are not financially compensated. Other things being equal, community care will appear more attractive than institutional care when informal care is not costed.

Measurement of time devoted to non-market activities

The first task is to identify how much time is being used or is being released as a consequence of treatment. Generally the focus is on patients and other household members but the issues and methods are as relevant to the unpaid contributions of others, such as the time of volunteers contributing to community-based projects in low-income countries, especially health promotion interventions. Two main methods can be used to collect data: interviews and diaries. Interviews may be susceptible to recall bias. For example, longer inputs of time are more easily remembered than shorter time inputs. It may be possible to collect reliable data for the past two weeks but the further back someone is asked to recall, the poorer the accuracy of the data. Diaries may be a more accurate means of capturing the time spent on non-market activities, particularly where the time input is variable. However, the keeping of a diary is clearly a greater imposition than is a single interview.

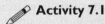 **Activity 7.1**

The measurement challenges are not all associated with the difficulties of accurately recalling events. What other problems do you think might arise in trying to identify the amount of time and effort an informal carer provides?

 Feedback

Frequently, caring is hard to separate from usual activities. For example, helping someone with their shopping while doing your own will require additional time but how much additional time? Laundry and food preparation activities may similarly be characterized by an element of joint production. This is an example of the problem of attribution. The aim is to capture changes in resource use as a consequence of the intervention.

As there was with productivity gains, there is an issue of perspective. Should all foregone activities be valued? For example, foregone leisure time undeniably has a value to the individual but it does not follow that it must be included in an assessment of how to allocate scarce health care resources. Whether or not it should will be determined by the perspective of the analysis. Given a societal perspective it will be included. Given a health service perspective it will be excluded.

Valuation of carers' time

One important missing market price is the cost of the time of volunteers, family members and others who often provide care. There is no readily identifiable market price for such activity, however, these inputs certainly have an opportunity cost in that time is a scarce resource like any other. A number of different methods have been proposed for valuing volunteer or informal carers' time. Three of these are reviewed by Brouwer *et al.* (2001).

- Value the output of the carer in terms of its market price, that is, the amount that it would cost to employ someone to undertake these activities. For example, in the case of planning and preparing meals, one extreme would be to value the part that involves planning at the wage rate of a dietician and that of cooking at the wage rate of a chef. Generally, this would provide an overestimate in that the carer is probably not performing these tasks to a similar level to that of a professional. Thus the alternative of what it would cost to employ an individual to supply all of the services is generally preferred.
- The productivity loss of the family member or other carer might be identified by considering what the unpaid worker could have earned had they instead spent the time in paid employment. A related notion, which might yield a different value, is the minimum amount that a person would require in order to take paid employment rather than spend their time providing care.
- Finally let the value depend on the nature of the time lost – what type of activity was displaced? A threefold classification of time has been proposed. Time spent on informal care could come from paid work time, unpaid work time or leisure time. Under this approach the amount of time displaced from each of the categories is identified and valued accordingly. Paid work time would be valued by the wage after deductions for tax. Unpaid work time is valued by estimating how much it would have been necessary to pay someone else to provide the informal care. Finally, it is proposed that changes in leisure time be reflected in quality of life measurements rather than measured in money terms.

Because of the many challenges involved in valuing non-market activities, the value placed on time is an important variable to examine in a sensitivity analysis (which you will learn about in Chapters 14 and 15).

✏ Activity 7.2

Table 7.2 compares methods for valuing the loss of time due to malaria by applying the methods and assumptions used by different authors to a common dataset. The notes below the table provide some details regarding these methods.

1   From the information presented try to explain the differences in results.

Table 7.2 Comparison of methods for valuing loss of time due to malaria

Study	Method	Total (Rs in 1993)	Per fully recovered patient
Attanayake et al.[1]	Output-related method	83 549	243
Sharma et al.[2]	Mean daily income	321 156	934
Asenso-Okyere and Dzator[3]	Average wage rate	155 975	453
Shepard et al.[4]	Daily output per adult	112 171	326
Ettling et al.[5]	Average income per day	84 500	246
Jayawardane[6]	Average wage rate	64 575	188
Sauerborn et al.[7]	Daily output per adult	16 608	48

Source: Attanayake et al. (2000)

1 Actual lost income and time spent covering for others valued at the average wage rate for manual labour. Lost agricultural output valued at local market prices. Time losses of economically inactive patients and those involved in housework not included.
2 Mean daily income of the household head was multiplied by the mean man days lost by a patient irrespective of age-gender categories. No emphasis was given for time lost to caring for patients.
3 Days lost by economically active adult patients including those who were between 11 and 17 years (if they work) were taken into consideration. Age-gender specific wage rates were used for valuing days lost. It was assumed that sick children were cared for by an adult female and therefore the adult female wage rate was used in valuing the time spent by carers. Only fully disabled days were used in this calculation.
4 Daily output per adult was estimated taking all economic activities into consideration. For adults, duration of the illness time, including partially disabled days, was multiplied by their average daily output. For children 30% of their duration of illness was taken as the time spent by adults caring for them and average adult daily output was used for valuation. Both men and women were treated equally in valuing loss of time.
5 Average income per household was used to estimate average income per adult. Treating all household members above 10 years as adults. Partially disabled days were treated as 'less work' days and valued as one-half of a lost workday. 'Working days' lost just for the purpose of caring for children under 10 years were valued using average daily adult income. The total number of 'working days' lost by carers was deducted from the total number of fully disabled days lost by children and the difference was considered as 'less work' days valued at half of daily income.
6 The days lost by fully recovered male household heads and the days spent by them caring for the other patients of the household were multiplied by the male average wage rate. The time loss of all other patients was not taken into consideration. Calculations were confined to the households where the head was infected with 'malaria' and fully recovered but not for the whole sample. In estimating the cost per patient, total cost of the household heads was divided by the total number of patients of the whole sample.
7 Daily output per adult was estimated taking all economic activities into consideration. Level of the severity of illness was used in valuing the loss of time: i.e. for adults one day for mild illness and five days for severe illness. One third of each of these time losses was applied for children below 15 years old. Both men and women were treated equally in valuing loss of time.

2 Identify what information you would ideally use to estimate the indirect costs of malaria.

Feedback

1 An important consideration is which household members are included in the calculation. Studies also differ with respect to how partially disabled days are treated. Time losses may be valued on an individual basis or using average values for groups. Some studies focus on time lost while others also consider lost agricultural output.

2 This is another question where differences of opinion are clearly possible. Your answer should clearly indicate what choices you are making with respect to which household members should be included. As it is information that you would ideally use it is likely that you will want individual data wherever possible rather than relying on averages. It is also likely that you would wish to distinguish between fully disabled days and partially disabled days.

The relative importance of the indirect costs discussed in this chapter varies widely. In some circumstances, particularly in low-income countries, these costs can be substantial relative to the direct costs of health care. For example, one of the studies of the costs of malaria in Sri Lanka referred to in Table 7.2 found that three-quarters of the total costs were made up of indirect costs (Attanayake *et al.* 2000). As a result, if these non-market consequences are ignored, the costs of different interventions and the benefits from successful treatment may be greatly underestimated. However, just which activities should be included is debatable. Data collection difficulties are if anything more formidable than in the case of the direct costs of health care since few data are ever routinely collected. There are a range of methods for valuing the non-market resource consequences which generally attempt to anticipate the values that would be generated if the relevant market existed.

Summary

You have seen how the economic impact of health care outside the health care sector can be identified, measured and valued. These are essential to consider if you are evaluating the economic impact of health care on society rather than just on health services. Judgements must be made as to exactly which resources to include in any given evaluation.

References

Attanayake N, Fox-Rushby J and Mills A (2000) Household costs of 'malaria' morbidity: a study in Matale district, Sri Lanka. *Tropical Medicine and International Health* 5:595–606, (www.blackwell-synergy.com).

Brouwer W, Rutten F and Koopmanschap M (2001) Costing in economic evaluations, in M Drummond and A McGuire (eds) *Economic evaluation in health care: merging theory with practice.* Oxford: Oxford University Press.

Dolan P and Olsen JA (2002) *Distributing health care: economic and ethical issues* Oxford. Oxford University Press.

SECTION 3

Measuring and valuing consequences

8 | Approaches to measuring health and life

Overview

In order to know whether a health intervention provides value for money you need to know how much, of what, is produced and how valuable it is. You have already learnt about identifying all the impacts of the intervention. In this chapter you will move on to deciding how to quantify the outcomes of interest and how to value the measured changes. This chapter recognizes the broad spectrum of measures available, justifies the criteria on which an economist would choose to select measures and compares the measures. The chapter ends by reflecting on the role of translation for measurement of health internationally.

Learning objectives

After working through this chapter, you will be able to:

- **explain how conceptions of health vary and how this affects whether health care interventions are considered effective and therefore efficient**
- **explain which type of outcome measures are most suitable for use in economic evaluation**
- **calculate changes in life expectancy using life tables**
- **provide a justified choice of health measures to evaluate the effectiveness and efficiency of a health care intervention**
- **reflect on some of the challenges of using existing health status measures in new cultural settings**

Key terms

Dimension/multidimensional One or many aspects (to health).

Effect size The average change in health scoring divided by either the standard deviation or baseline of change score.

Health index One number (usually between 0 and 1) that summarizes the relative value of several dimensions of health.

Health profile A graphical summary of each dimension of health measured.

Health-related quality of life How a person's health affects their ability to carry out functional activities and well-being according to their own subjective opinion.

Morbidity This has two meanings: being ill and the illness rate of a population.

Mortality This has two meanings: being mortal and the death rate of a population.

Psychometrics The science of psychological measurement.

Reliability The extent to which an instrument produces consistent results.

Responsiveness The ability of a measure to detect a clinically meaningful change.

Scenario A brief description of a state of health.

Validity The extent to which an indicator measures what it intends to measure.

Weighting (scoring, scale) A measure of relative value or the act of giving the relative value such as assigning a number or physical mark on a defined continuum.

Conceptions of health

Any measure of health is rooted (implicitly or explicitly) in beliefs about what health is. However, there are many different views about this. Vego-Franco (2002) has suggested eleven definitions of health:

- balance in bodily humours (Galenic view);
- blood, phlegm, yellow and black bile;
- biological and psychological security;
- harmonious functioning of organs and bodily systems;
- a life of restraint to preserve harmony; harmony with the gods and protection from evil spirits;
- interaction between internal and external environments;
- internal homeostasis (complex balance of cells, fluids and tissues) and external homeostasis (harmonious balance that keeps society together);
- state of complete physical, mental and social well-being, and not merely the absence of disease or infirmity (the WHO aspirational goal);
- the absence of disease; the balance of competing life forces (the *yin* and *yang* of Chinese medicine); and
- the harmony of wind, fire and water (Ayurvedic medicine).

The way health is thought about is affected by personal experience. For example, the views of lay people and of health care professionals differ, as do those of older people and teenagers.

 Activity 8.1

What do you think health is? Make a list of what you think it does and does not include. It may help to think about what you consider good and bad health to be.

 Feedback

There are no right answers to this question as it is a matter of personal belief. However, it is important to recognize how you think about health yourself because this will influence which measures you think are appropriate.

You are reading this book in English. The authors of this chapter are English and Scottish and, whilst predominantly working in the UK, have extensive experience working and living in a variety of countries. All these facts affect the way that each of us will think about health. It is therefore relevant to think about the way in which the English word 'health' might be used as this will reflect ways in which people think and therefore contribute to international debates on public health.

Allen *et al.* (1997) suggested several usages of the English word 'health', including:

1 Health is the absence of bodily (and possibly psychological) malfunction. This is a reductive notion of health. It treats the English word 'health' as a word that, like any word, can be translated. It takes a limited biomedical meaning and applies it universally. It implies that local ways of seeing the world are relevant only in so far as they relate to clinically observable phenomena.
2 Health is represented by the resonance of local equivalencies for the connotations of the English word 'health'. This explores the context and use of connotations of the local words for the English word 'health'. It assumes that all humans have a certain range of concerns about their existence.
3 Health as reflected in the overlap of local ways of seeing the world with ways of seeing implied (to English speakers) by the word 'health'. This is an extension of the previous conception. However, it accepts that some people may have either no or little understanding of an arena of experience that corresponds to the word 'health'.

 Activity 8.2

If usages 1 or 3 above reflected your view, how might this affect:

a) the choice of measurement instrument selected or developed
b) the type of health intervention shown to be effective
c) the type of health intervention shown to be efficient?

 Feedback

a) Using conception 1 is more likely to result in choosing a measure based on the functioning of mind and body. Using conception 3 is more likely to result in a measure of health that is broader than biomedical measures, more specific to non-English speakers, and based on different philosophies.
b) A measure based on conception 1 is unlikely to show the full impact of a non-health care intervention or pick up the impact of interventions on social relationships and will therefore under-represent any value attached to such change. As measures based on usage 1 have a greater focus on physical change, interventions aimed at physical improvements are more likely to demonstrate effectiveness. Interventions shown to be effective are more likely to be provided and hence usage 1 is more likely to result in the provision of biomedical interventions. As usage 3 is broader, interventions that restore an individual to full physical health will only be shown to have a partial impact on overall health and are therefore less likely to be provided than an intervention that also improves social relations.

c) This answer is related to the point above, because if an intervention is not shown to be effective it cannot be efficient and an intervention that is less (more) effective, all other things being equal, will also be less (more) efficient.

Different conceptions of health affect the definition of health chosen, the choice of instrument for measuring outcomes and, therefore, the type of interventions recommended. Not surprisingly, given the variety of conceptions of health and range of diseases, there is a vast array of measurement tools. What is important to ask is which types of measure are useful for economic evaluation to inform the allocation of resources?

Characteristics of good measures for economic evaluations

The first important characteristic for any measure of health is that it can be used to compare changes across diseases and interventions. Consider the case of CEA. You know that CEA can be used to compare the costs and effects of alternative interventions for one disease. Why then is comparison important? Imagine that the cost of one intervention is higher but health outcomes are better compared with the other intervention. Should the more costly intervention be funded? In terms of resource allocation, you would need to know whether the additional health benefits are more or less expensive than with other interventions for other diseases. Therefore, even though an evaluation may focus on only one disease, the results need to be interpreted in a comparative way for resource allocation purposes.

The second requirement is that the health measures have a scale with interval properties. This is, first, because it is not enough to know that health has improved or declined – you need to know by how much it has changed. Second, changes in health need to be related to changes in expenditure and therefore scaled up and down. A scale can have binary, ordinal or cardinal properties. A binary variable has two options (e.g. being alive or dead or having a disease or not). People may prefer to be alive or not to have a disease but that is the extent to which preferences may be known. A scale with ordinal properties can be ranked from most to least preferred. An example would be asking people whether they like something 'not at all', 'a little', 'quite a bit', or 'a lot'. You would know that 'a little' is better than 'not at all' but not by *how much*. A cardinal scale could have either interval or ratio properties. Interval properties would mean that equal intervals existed between numbers (i.e. a move from 30 to 40 was the same size as a move from 20 to 30) but not make any assumption about the absolute size of numbers (i.e. interval scales could not state that the number represented by 40 was twice the size of 20). Scales that have a true zero point are able to compare the size of numbers (rather than just size of change) and are known as 'ratio scales'.

Activity 8.3

State whether the variables listed below have ratio, interval, ordinal or binary scales. Which variables might you be unsure about and why?

1   Years of life lived with arthritis.
2   Whether been ill in last month or not.
3   Temperature measured in degrees Celsius.
4   Money.
5   Feeling unhappy, happy, very happy or ecstatic.
6   The tastiness of soup (where people have made a mark somewhere on a straight
    line with one end labelled 'delicious' and the other end labelled 'disgusting').
7   Days spent in pain.

Feedback

Numbers 1, 4 and 7 are ratio scales because a true zero exists (e.g. no days in pain).
Numbers 3 and 6 have interval properties, as a true zero does not exist; the zero on a
Celsius scale is not no temperature (in fact it is 273° using the Kelvin temperature
scale). Number 5 is ordinal and number 2 binary. Number 6 might raise most doubt.
There is not a true zero here (you can imagine people having different views about
whether there is no taste) but you might want further evidence to check that people
really are using it as an equal interval scale and not as a ranked scale.

The third most important characteristic is that health measures reflect preferences,
either of individual patients or the general public. This characteristic derives from
consumer theory that is built on a structuring of desires by consumers for alternative combinations of goods and services. Consumers weigh up the benefits of
options and compare these with the costs before making a purchase (whether in
money or time spent accessing a service). Considering consumer preferences under
conditions of risk and uncertainty can incorporate the uncertainties inherent in
disease and health care.

A second set of characteristics derived from principles of psychometrics (the quantification and measurement of psychological phenomena) is important in certain
circumstances. These characteristics are summarized below (Brazier *et al.* 2001):

- *Reliability*: the ability of a measure to produce repeated results from an
  unchanged population with limited random error. It is evaluated by comparing
  results from repeated tests over short time periods and from data collected by
  multiple interviewers.
- *Validity*: the extent to which a measure captures what it purports to measure. In
  health measurement there is no gold standard and therefore validity is measured indirectly using content (the appropriateness of items within an instrument) and construct validity (the extent to which results correlate with other
  indicators, measures or concepts of interest in accordance with expectations).
- *Practicality*: the measure should be acceptable to respondents and ethics committees as well as being easy to administer, score and interpret findings.
  Response rates and quantity of missing data is one way that acceptability is
  assessed quantitatively.
- *Responsiveness*: a measure should be able to detect change in health status over
  time and be able to detect a clinically or socially meaningful change. A com-

monly used approach is to calculate the 'effect size', which is the difference between the mean baseline and mean follow-up scores divided by the standard deviation of the baseline scores. For example, if mean symptom scores at baseline and follow-up were 14.5 and 8.5 respectively and the standard deviation at baseline were 9.1, the effect size would be: $(14.5–8.5)/9.1 = 0.66$. A measure with an effect size of 0.2 is considered fairly unresponsive whereas an effect size of 0.8 is responsive.

 Activity 8.4

Does a measure with a big effect size indicate the value or importance of a change in health?

 Feedback

The effect size indicates the relative size of the signal to 'noise' in the data. A large effect size does not indicate a larger value because the value of change has not been assessed. If people were asked to value changes in health, a very different mean and standard deviation might occur.

Types of health measures available

There are many ways of measuring the impact of health care interventions on health (see Table 8.1). You will now learn about each approach and compare how each measures up to the requirements of an economic evaluation.

Table 8.1 Types of health measure

- Mortality
  - Deaths averted
  - Life years gained
- Morbidity
  - Prevalence and incidence of a disease
  - Clinical measures of impairment (e.g. X-ray findings, blood levels)
- Disease-specific measures
  - Disease profiles (e.g. chronic respiratory distress questionnaire)
  - Disease indices (e.g. Arthritis Impact Measurement Scale (AIMS))
- Generic health measures
  - Health profiles (e.g. Nottingham Health Profile (NHP), 100 question WHO quality of life measure (WHOQOL 100))
  - Health indices
    - Non-preference-based (e.g. Short Form–36 (SF-36))
    - Preference based (e.g. EuroQol 5 dimensional measure (EQ5D), Health Utilities Index (HUI), Quality of Well-Being Index (QWB))

Mortality

The most frequently used measure of health today is death rates and the duration of life. It is important to represent any change in survival of a population over time from an intervention, particularly in parts of the world where mortality rates are higher at younger ages.

Life tables provide a comprehensive measure of the impact of mortality on life expectancy (LE). They present data for a hypothetical population born at the same time who are then subject to age-specific mortality rates, usually in periods of one year. Life tables can be calculated for general populations in each country as well as population subgroups (e.g. age, sex, race) and cause (e.g. cardiovascular disease).

 Activity 8.5

Table 8.2 gives an example of a life table. By assuming a distribution of when deaths occur within a year (e.g. equally), the total person years lived at any age can be calculated.

1 Calculate the probability of survival from age 2 to 5.

2 If 99,180 survive to the age of 6 and 99,163 survive to age 7, and the value of $T_{(x)}$ is 7,229,477, calculate the expectation of life for age 5–6.

3 If a new intervention reduces the mortality rate amongst 0–2 year olds by 30% whilst all other mortality rates remain the same, how many life years would be saved? (NB the new $T_{(x)}$ would be 7,725,884 for 0–1 yrs and 7,626,616 for 1–2 yrs).

 Feedback

a) Divide the number of survivors at age 5 (99,200) by the number of survivors at age 2 (99,303) = 0.99896.

b) 72.9.

c) Step 1: The mortality rate for the 0–1 group is 0.00488 and for the 1–2 yr group is 0.00033.
Step 2: Person years lived between ages 2–3 is 99,580.
Step 3: The total life years for the 2 age groups (7,725,884 + 7,626,616 = 15,352,500), subtracting the previous number of life years (15,352,187) you get 313 additional life years per 100,000 population from a 30% mortality reduction in ages 0–2 yrs.

To calculate the impact on life expectancy after introducing a new treatment, the information required would be cause-specific life expectancy, prevalence of the disease, relative risk of mortality prior to the treatment and the risk reduction following treatment. However, in practice these are not always available and therefore you have to seek approximate changes in mortality. A commonly used

Table 8.2 Life table for the 0–5 yrs: United States, 2002

Age	Probability of dying between ages x to x + 1	Number surviving to age x	Number dying between ages x to x + 1	Person-years lived between ages x to x + 1	Total number of person-years lived above age x	Expectation of life at age x
	$q_{(x)}$	$l_{(x)}$	$d_{(x)}$	$L_{(x)}$	$T_{(x)}$	$e_{(x)}$
0–1	0.00697	100,000	697	99,389	7,725,787	77.3
1–2	0.000472	99,303	47	99,279	7,626,399	76.8
2–3	0.000324	99,256	32	99,240	7,527,119	75.8
3–4	0.000239	99,224	24	99,212	7,427,879	74.9
4–5	0.000203	99,200	20	99,190	7,328,667	73.9

Source: http://www.cdc.gov/nchs/products/pubs/pubd/lftbls/lftbls.htm (accessed 23/01/05)

alternative is the Declining Exponential Approximation of Life Expectancy (DEALE) method that requires only estimates of baseline life expectancy and the excess mortality rate μ from the particular cause of death (DEALE = $1/(\mu+1/LE)$) (Beck *et al.* 1982). However, the method can underestimate LE in younger patients and this is one of the reasons for adopting alternative approaches to survival analysis.

Morbidity

Morbidity is most often reported as prevalence (the number of people in a given population affected with a particular disease at a point in time) and incidence rates (the number of new cases of a disease or condition in a specific population over a given period of time). The main problem with morbidity rates is that they only indicate presence of a disease and tell us nothing about the duration or impact on a person's life. Whilst clinical measures such as the results from X-rays and blood tests give an indication of the severity of disease, they tell us nothing about what impact this has on a patient's ability and how they feel.

Disease- or condition-specific instruments

Disease-specific measures focus on changes in severity of symptoms related to specific diseases or conditions and sometimes on the types of impact these have on patients' quality of life. These measures differ not only by disease but also within disease groups. They can consist of single items – for example, one question about pain or many questions about the impact of disease on many aspects of life (Bowling 2001).

Comparing the Arthritic Impairment Measurement Scale (AIMS) with the Chronic Respiratory Distress Questionnaire (CRDQ) highlights the diversity of measures. The AIMS was developed to measure the health status of people with arthritic diseases following criticisms that existing instruments took too narrow a view of health and at the same time did not include issues of importance to patients with arthritis (e.g. dexterity, bathing/dressing and pain). The CRDQ was developed because generic health measures were considered too insensitive to changes in patients with respiratory disease. The AIMS is a self-administered questionnaire with 45 questions grouped into nine dimensions, with each dimension scored between 0–10. For example, dexterity is assessed by enquiring as to a person's ability to write with a pen or turn a key in a lock. The CRDQ is an interview where patients are asked to identify five activities most important to them that produce most breathlessness and identify the impact of the disease followed by a series of questions about fatigue, emotional function and feelings of control over the disease in the last two weeks. Scores are produced for the feelings but not summed.

Generic health status measures

Generic health status measures are:

"designed to be broadly applicable across types and severities of disease, across different medical treatments or health interventions, and across demographic and cultural subgroups. These measures are also designed to summarize a spectrum of core concepts of health and quality of life that apply to many different diseases, impairments, conditions, patients and populations." (Patrick and Erickson 1993)

Generic measures exist as profiles or indices. Health profiles present different dimensions of health separately whereas health indices provide a single summary index score. The significant advantage of representing the multidimensional concept of health as an index value is that a unique solution for comparisons of health gain across interventions, diseases and populations exists. There are two ways of aggregating scores to produce the single value: those that do and those that do not account for people's preferences.

If index scores for generic measures are created without accounting for preferences, a higher or lower number does not necessarily mean that people value the state more or less. Indeed, research has shown that health status measures and preference-based measures are, at best, only moderately correlated (Revicki and Kaplan 1993). Also, index scores that have no reference point within the instrument to death or perfect health cannot be used to combine changes in quality and quantity of life because there is no way of linking, comparing or trading off these different aspects of health.

✎ **Activity 8.6**

From the graphs showing health profile scores in Figure 8.1, work out whether the health of this group of patients has improved with treatment and justify your answer.

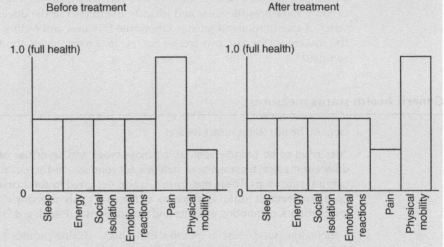

Figure 8.1 Health profile scores before and after treatment
Source: LSHTM

↻ **Feedback**

There is no impact of treatment on four dimensions and, although pain has worsened, physical mobility has improved. As a health profile does not combine scores it is not clear whether overall health has improved or which option is preferred. If dimension scores were weighted equally, there would be no overall difference in health before and after the intervention. If pain were given a higher weight, the overall result would be a decrease in health (scores closer to zero indicate worse health). If the weight were a preference weight then people would prefer not to have the treatment.

Table 8.3 compares a selection of generic measures. These can be short and simple (most only take around 10–15 minutes to complete) and can be administered in a variety of ways (e.g. interview, questionnaire, over the telephone). Health indices tend to have fewer dimensions (and occasionally very few questions) and this is why indices are less responsive to change than health profiles. Only one health index has been developed internationally (the EQ5D) and only one health profile has been developed within low- and middle-income countries from the outset (WHOQOL-100).

Table 8.4 compares different types of measure using the categorisation from Table 8.1 with the characteristics of good measures for economic evaluations (from the second section of this chapter). It shows which instruments meet the criteria and

Table 8.3 Selected generic health status and quality of life measures

Name of measure	Dimensions	Number of questions	Where originally developed	Type of measure
WHOQOL 100	Physical, psychological, levels of independence, social relationship, environment, spiritual domain	100	Bangkok, Bath, Madras, Melbourne, Panama, Seattle, St Petersburg, Tilburg, Zagreb, Zimbabwe	Profile
NHP	Part 1: energy, social isolation, pain, physical mobility, sleep, emotional reactions	38	In and around Nottingham and Derbyshire, UK	Profile
SF-36	Physical health (physical functioning, role-physical, bodily pain, general health) and one for mental health (vitality, social functioning, role-emotional, mental health)	36	Boston, Chicago, Los Angeles	Profile and non-preference index, now with preference index (SF6D)
QWB	Mobility, physical activity, social activity + 27 symptoms/problems (e.g. pain, fever, loss of consciousness)	50	New York State and San Diego, California	Preference-based index
EQ5D	Mobility, self-care, usual activities, pain/discomfort, anxiety/depression	5	York, West and Central London (UK), Rotterdam (Netherlands), Lund (Sweden), Helsinki (Finland), Oslo (Norway)	Preference-based index

Source: Adapted from Fox-Rushby and Parker (1995)

WHO QOL = WHO quality of life
NHP = Nottingham Health Profile
SF-36 = Short Form 36
QWB = Quality of Well Being
EQSD = European Quality of Life – 5 dimensions

Table 8.4 Comparison of types of health status measures using economic and psychometric criteria

	Economic criteria			Psychometric criteria			
	Comparability across disease	Interval scale?	Individual preference-based scoring?	Reliable	Valid	Practical	Responsive
Mortality	Yes	Yes	No	Depends on surveillance system			No
Morbidity	No	No	No	Depends on surveillance system			No
Disease-specific measures	No	Yes and no	No	Yes and no	Yes and no	Yes and no	Yes
Generic health profiles	Yes	No	No	Yes	Yes	Yes	More than preference-based indices, less than disease-specific measures
Generic indices (non-preference)	Yes	No	No	Yes	Yes	Yes	More than preference-based indices, less than disease-specific measures
Generic indices (preference based)	Yes	Yes	Yes	Yes (unless very many health states)	Yes	Yes	Often not

which do not. The table shows that only health indices using preference weights are completely compatible with economic evaluation, even though they are often not very responsive to change, particularly marginal changes in randomized trials. One of the options open to you is to use a health index with more health states, with the possibility of being better able to discriminate between small changes. The Health Utilities Index (HUI) developed in Canada has 972,000 health states compared with the potential 243 of the EQ5D. However, the reliability of values for the HUI has been questioned as the estimation of values rests on relatively few data.

Table 8.3 shows that the second most useful measure is change in mortality, even though it is a very restrictive view of health. There is little to choose between the remaining measures using economic criteria. The main limitation of disease-based measures is being unable to compare health across disease. The psychometric criteria suggest that generic rather than disease-based measures are likely to be more reliable and valid (although this will depend on the particular disease-specific instrument selected for comparison). Indeed, there has been a concerted effort to develop valid and reliable generic scales and this has encouraged such widespread use that population norms now exist for several questionnaires.

Is there any value to non-preference based measures of health status in economic evaluation? Can disease measures play any role other than for specific disease-based evaluations? Among several possibilities, Brazier *et al.* (2001) suggested that valuation of HRQL for use in economic appraisal requires a valid description of health and that both health- and disease-specific profiles can help with this. One way is to help describe any changes measured in 'scenarios', which are the basis for much of the valuation techniques described in the next chapter. The more meaningful those scenarios are to those providing values, the more reliable and valid the valuations are likely to be.

The role of translation in generic health status measures

Multidimensional generic measures of HRQL are used across the world. Generic measures are being used in an increasing number of countries and so instruments are being translated. However, there is now widespread concern that it is inappropriate to simply ask a 'fluent' friend to translate an instrument prior to its use. Therefore there are increasingly sophisticated guidelines on how to ensure good quality translations (see Table 8.5) and a move by regulatory agencies to control translation processes.

The advantage of translation is that existing instruments can become available in new languages relatively quickly. However, some have criticized this process as being rooted in an absolutist view of the world (Herdman *et al.* 1998), with health treated as if it were an 'objective truth'. Also, the increasing sophistication in translations means the process may not be quick and may end with a decision that an instrument is not appropriate for the target culture. In addition, when translators have sought to change questionnaires that translate badly, the original developers of instruments have not always agreed to the changes. Not only may the developers have spent over ten years developing the instrument but they may also draw on arguments to suggest that changing questions would mean results are not comparable across countries.

Table 8.5 One set of steps recommended for translating HRQL instruments

Step 1 (forward step)
- Contact author of original instrument
- Produce several forward translations
- Ensure translators are based in the target, not source, country
- Consensus meeting for all those producing forward translations to agree one version

Step 2 (quality review)
- Back-translate the consensus version of forward translation (to detect any errors and changes in meaning)
- Rate the quality of the forward translation (judge conceptual equivalence with the original, clarity and use of the familiar/colloquial language)

Step 3 (pre-testing)
- Ask monolingual lay panel to review translation
- Bilingual lay panel to compare translation and original version
- Test translation on future users ensuring range of relevant ages, gender, socioeconomic background etc.

Step 4 (international harmonization if a multi-country study)
- Bring together translators from each target language to focus on and discuss the main 'problem areas' of the questionnaire

Step 5 (documentation)
- Document the translation process giving evidence to the quality of the translation process and validity of future cross-country comparisons

Step 6 (re-weighting/scoring)
- Consider the need to re-weight scoring mechanisms

Source: Acquadro *et al.* (1996)

Arguments about the cross-cultural comparability of HRQL questionnaires should be based on consideration of the degree to which questionnaires are equivalent. However, Bowden and Fox-Rushby (2003) showed that even in Japan, where translation has been most evident, little research has focused on the extent to which concepts of health, and its constituent parts represented in instruments, are shared between source and target language groups.

Should translation not be considered appropriate, your options are to: choose another measure, noting the limitations and likely impact on results; measure activities rather than outcome; use an existing model (or develop a new one) to predict the relationship between activities and outcomes; or develop a new measure. Brooks (1995) helpfully outlined broad approaches for developing measures with large and small budgets but you should be aware of the commitments and requirements of developing new measures prior to embarking on such a journey.

🖉 Activity 8.7

The Ministry of Health in Heretica is developing a call for proposals to evaluate the cost-effectiveness of a new method for cataract surgery alongside a randomized trial. They would like to consider the impact on outcomes.

1 What types of outcome measures would you advise them to consider and why?
2 How would you expect applicants to decide on an appropriate measure?

Feedback

1 If there is more than one expected use of results (e.g. effectiveness of surgery and resource allocation) then it is pertinent to use more than one outcome measure, but there should be an indication of which is the primary outcome measure as this should be used in determining the sample size. The following could be included:

- mortality: impact on life years gained, as sight has an impacts on mortality over time
- condition-specific measures: to detect change, these might include a range of clinical indicators (e.g. sight tests), symptom measures and condition-specific health status measures that relate sight to functioning or other aspects of health
- generic measures: this would allow comparison of results with other interventions. Given the variety of instruments, this should include those developed or used among those with sight difficulties and ideally provide an index value

2 Depending on the size of the budget, this would include:

- reviewing the use of existing HRQL measures in assessing the impact of cataract surgery (as a minimum noting evidence on reliability, validity and sensitivity as well as types of people among which it had been used, main findings and whether or not used in Heretica)
- to ascertain which of the potentially relevant instruments have been translated for use in Heretica, noting the quality of the translation
- some process of consultation with Ministry of Health officials, other health professionals and patients
- expected use of results
- piloting and pre-testing of selected instruments

Summary

You have learnt about the different conceptions of health and how these may affect the type of health measures you use in an economic evaluation. You went on to learn about the characteristics of a good measure and the advantages and limitations of generic and disease-specific measures.

References

Acquadro C et al. (1996) Language and translation issues, in D Spilker (ed.) Quality of life and pharmacoeconomics in clinical trials, 2nd edn. Philadelphia: Lippincot-Raven.
Allen T et al. (1997) Conceptions of health in quality of life research. Quality of Life Research 6(7/8):614.
Beck JR, Pauker SG, Gotleib JE, Klein K and Kassirer JP (1982) A convenient approximation of life expectancy (the 'DEALE'): use in medical decision-making. The American Journal of Medicine 73:889–97.
Bowden A and Fox-Rushby JA (2003) A systematic and critical review of the process of translation and adaptation of generic health-related quality of life measures in Africa, Asia, Eastern Europe, the Middle East and South America. Social Science and Medicine 57(7):1289–306.
Bowling A (2001) Measuring disease, 2nd edn. Buckingham: Open University Press.

Brazier J, Deverill M, Green C, Harper R and Booth A (2001) *A review of the use of health status measures in economic evaluation health technology assessment*, www.ncchta.org/fullmono/mon309.pdf.

Brooks R (1995) *Health status: A perspective on change*. Basingstoke: Macmillan.

Fox-Rushby J and Parker M, 'Culture and the measurement of health-related quality of life,' European Journal of Applied Psychology/Revue Europeene de Psychologie Appliquee, 45(4): 257–263, Elsevier. Reprinted by permission of Les Editions du Centre de Psychologie Appliquée.

Herdman M, Fox-Rushby J and Badia X (1998) A model of equivalence in the cultural adaptation of HRQL instruments: the universalist approach. *Quality of Life Research* 7:323–55.

Patrick D and Erickson P (1993) *Health status and health policy: allocating resources to health care*. Oxford: Oxford University Press.

Revicki DA and Kaplan RM (1993) Relationship between psychometric and utility-based approaches to the measurement of health-related quality of life. *Quality of Life Research* 2:477–87.

Vego-Franco L (2002) Ideas, creencia y percepiones acerca de las salud (Ideas, beliefs and perceptions about health: a historical account). *Salud Public Mex*, 44:258–65.

Further reading

Bowling A (2004) *Measuring health: a review of quality of life measurement scales*, 2nd edn. Maidenhead: Open University Press.

http://bmj.bmjjournals.com/collections/statsbk explains the calculation of survival curves.

The International Society of Quality of Life Research (ISOQOL) promotes the rigorous investigation of health-related quality of life measurement from conceptualization to application and practice. See www.isoqol.org/ for further details.

9

Valuing changes in health using non-monetary approaches

Overview

In this chapter you will learn about a range of techniques developed to elicit utility values for health states. This allows the different components of health to be represented as a single number that captures the way that people feel components of health have value in relation to each other. Because improvements in quality of life are only part of health improvement, this chapter also considers other approaches to combining quality and quantity of life in a single index value.

Learning objectives

After working through this chapter, you will be able to:

- **compare and contrast alternative approaches for eliciting non-monetary values of health**
- **calculate the impact of a health care intervention in terms of QALYs gained and DALYs averted**
- **consider the pros and cons of QALYs and DALYs**

Key terms

Health state scenario A description of several (usually three to seven) dimensions of a hypothetical person's health.

Observed/stated preferences What consumers reveal they want through actions or what they say they want.

Preferences This assumes a real or imagined choice between at least two options that can be ranked.

Pre-scored questionnaire A questionnaire that can help categorize the state of health dimensions and then use existing data to value the state.

Introduction

It is in the area of valuation that health economics has had the greatest contribution to the development of outcome assessment. The aim of valuing anything is to estimate how desirable something is – to decide its worth or, as economists say, utility. Research has centred both on monetary and non-monetary methods, with the majority of recent research concentrating on the latter. Thus valuation approaches in the health sector have been more often applied as CUA rather than CBA.

The advantage of pursuing HRQL beyond the stage of measurement is that different characteristics of health can be valued on a single scale and therefore compared. This approach has been incorporated into explicit decision-making, for example use of DALYs by the World Bank and the Quality of Well Being (QWB) scale by Oregon State in the USA.

In this chapter you will first consider two approaches to creating index values for health status: scenario-based approaches and pre-scored questionnaires, both of which are explained in turn with examples. You will then move on to see how to combine changes in the index value for health with changes in quantity of life, which leads to descriptions, activities and a comparison between QALYs and DALYs. The chapter ends by considering what characteristics, other than a health states alone, might affect values given to health states.

Methods for creating indices according to preferences

In Chapter 8 you learnt about the possibility that information from health- and disease-specific profiles could be used to create scenarios. Therefore, you begin the valuation process with this step. Scenarios are brief descriptions of a state of health. Here are two examples:

Scenario 1 One year ago you were told that you had schistosomiasis. Every three months or so you have had a very high fever. You often have little energy and it is difficult to fulfil all your farming duties although you struggle on with the easier ones. At times your children have to take time off school to help you. You often have diarrhoea and are unhappy about your skin having itchy blotches. You also have a cough that just seems to stay. You have seriously wondered about the cause of this illness, so much so that relations with some of your neighbours have soured.

Scenario 2 One year ago you experienced several dizzy spells over a period of two months. Your work was not affected but you did ask your spouse to drive the car, as you were always worrying about when it would happen. Six months later you began to feel dizzy again and have fainted once or twice a month. You also feel breathless when doing any form of exercise and have had some palpitations. Now you are unable to operate any kind of machinery. You worry about passing out and find yourself checking silently that someone is always around in case anything happens.

✎ Activity 9.1

Considering these two scenarios:

1   What aspects of health are covered in each?
2   What other kinds of information are given?

3 Did you think about what might have caused the description in Scenario 2? If so, what did you consider and how do you think that would affect people's perception of the severity of that disease state?

4 What else do you think could have been included?

5 Which scenario made more sense to you personally and why?

6 If you wanted to develop scenarios for a different disease, how might you go about developing them?

Feedback

1 There are different aspects of health included in each scenario. Scenario 1 includes symptoms (e.g. fever, diarrhoea, itchy skin, cough), ability to do activities (e.g. duties, farming), support given (e.g. by children taking time off school to help), feelings (concerns about the cause, unhappiness about blotchy skin) as well as beliefs of causality (e.g. that an illness might have been caused by something neighbours had done). Scenario 2 includes symptoms (e.g. dizziness, fainting, palpitations, breathlessness), ability to do activities (e.g. ability to operate machinery, exercise), and worries (e.g. about fainting).

2 There are several references to different time periods. Both scenarios also give an indication of how life is lived: the first refers to farming and ability to pull children out of school to help when needed; the second refers to both men and women driving cars and the opportunity to move between manual and desk jobs.

3 There is no right answer to this question. Scenario 2 might have referred to asthma, panic attacks or a cardiac problem. In fact, it describes someone with a cardiac pacemaker, which shows how respondents often interpret information differently. One solution is to label the disease in question, which Scenario 1 did. However, it is known that labels themselves affect the way people think about health states and often not in the ways described in the scenario (e.g. thinking a health state is more or less serious). All these possibilities mean that if people are asked to place a value on a health state, they may be influenced by ideas other than those presented in the scenario and that values may be inflated or deflated.

4 Any number of other aspects of health such as impact on pain levels, general mobility, energy levels and harmony in relationships (see previous chapter for a fuller set of ideas) might have been included, depending on the conception of health underpinning the work.

5 Personal knowledge and likelihood of experience may affect valuations.

6 Different degrees of effort might be put into the construction of scenarios. They may be developed on the advice of a few experts (as with DALYs), from qualitative research with patients, from the results of health measurement or using existing health status measures. The most useful are those that can link health states to quantities of patients in that health state and who change from one health state to another.

Once descriptions of health have been drawn up, the aim is to value them and thus be able to value any changes between health states. One important question is whose values should be used? Options include the general population, health care professionals and patients. Research has shown that these groups give different values to the same health state and this can potentially affect which types of intervention are funded. The advantage of choosing either patients or professionals is that values are based on experience. Nevertheless, experience may differ from the written scenarios given and there may be a range of unidentified incentives behind answers. The advantage of choosing the general public is that decision-making is aimed at these groups and all may potentially benefit (or not) from a decision. The difficulty with approaching the general public is that they may find it difficult to imagine being in the health states described.

Methods for valuing health states

The variety of techniques available to assign values to health states is distinguished by whether questions are framed as certainty or uncertainty and whether choices between competing alternatives are made or not. Table 9.1 shows that only the standard gamble (SG) asks about choices with uncertain outcomes. All other approaches ask respondents to consider health states as if they occur with certainty. You will learn about the three approaches: the visual analogue scale (VAS), time trade-off (TTO) and the SG.

Table 9.1 Methods of measuring preferences

	Question framing	
Response method	Certainty (values)	Uncertainty (V-N utilities)
Scaling	• Rating scale • Category rating • Visual analogue scale • Ratio scale	–
Choice	• Time trade-off • Paired comparisons • Equivalence • Person trade-off	• Standard gamble

Source: Drummond *et al.* (1997)

Visual analogue scales

Sometimes the best way to begin to understand a measurement instrument is to complete it yourself and these valuation methods are no exception.

✎ Activity 9.2

1 Re-read the two health scenarios above and imagine what it would be like if you were in these states. In Figure 9.1, draw a line from each health state to somewhere on the scale to indicate how good or bad you think this state is.

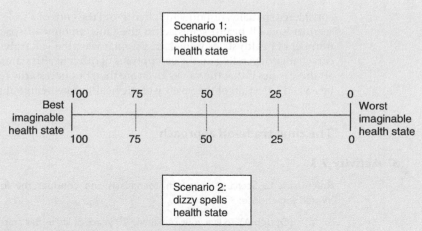

Figure 9.1 Placing health states on a VAS to indicate relative value

2   Calculate roughly what % level you placed health state scenario 1 and 2 at.
3   When people are asked to do this exercise, a range of values across the group is found. Why do you think this happens and what hypotheses might you use to test why differences occur?

 Feedback

1   There are no right answers. Your own opinion is valid.

2   If one of your lines is aimed at the centre, the % for that scenario would be 50%.

3   Some of the reasons are linked to difficulties in: likelihood of catching schistosomiasis; presence and age of children; needing to drive because living in a remote place; someone in family having asthma or cardiac disease; country in which living; awfulness of the health state. Many of these ideas (including others such as age, type of professional experience) could be turned into hypotheses and tested if appropriate data were collected.

Activity 9.2 demonstrated that it is possible to value very different health states on one scale and the advantages of VASs themselves: they are a practical, efficient and an easy to use method. As a results VASs have been used in many settings including laboratories, household interview surveys and self-completed questionnaires.

There are a number of disadvantages of a VAS. First, a zero score does not equal zero health (note the bottom of the scale was labelled 'worst imaginable health'). Therefore the scale does not have ratio properties and it is not possible to accept a score of 40 is twice that of 20. The EuroQol has used 'dead' both at the bottom of the scale and as a state to value in order to circumvent this problem but there is still debate about whether this confers ratio properties. At best such scales have equal interval properties, such that differences in 20 are equal across the scale. A VAS can also be considered spatially; respondents often avoid the ends of a scale and have also been seen to 'spread' health states across the same amount of space regardless of the number of health states valued. In a similar way, the value given to a health state can change depending on the descriptions of other health states. The problem with all these issues is that the values given are then not necessarily reliable and may not be a valid reflection of the severity of the health state being valued.

The time trade-off approach

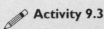 **Activity 9.3**

Refer back to Scenario 1 on schistosomiasis and consider the following question. Would you choose:

> (Option A) To live your remaining 20 years of life in this state
>   OR
> (Option B) To live in perfect health for 10 years?

If you chose Option A, go to question 1 below; if you chose Option B, go to question 2.

1   Would you choose:

> (Option A) To live for your remaining 15 years of life in this state
>   OR
> (Option B) To live in perfect health for 10 years?

Now work out how many years in this state would for you roughly equal 10 years lived in perfect health.

2   Would you choose:

> (Option A) To live for your remaining 30 years of life in this state
>   OR
> (Option B) To live in perfect health for 10 years

Now work out how many years in this state would for you roughly equal 10 years lived in perfect health.

3   Whichever option you chose, calculate the value you place on the health state described in Scenario 1 using the TTO. The preference score is calculated by x/t (where x is the time spent in perfect health and t is the time spent in the health state in the scenario).

4   Compare the TTO value with the value you gave to the same health state using the VAS completed in Activity 9.2.

 Feedback

If, for example, you consider that living for 15 years with schistosomiasis is roughly equal to 10 years in perfect health the preference value would be $10/15 = 0.67$.

Activity 9.3 shows that the TTO forces respondents into making a choice between having a shorter healthy life versus a longer life with ill health, as reflected in Figure 9.2.

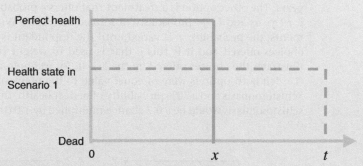

Figure 9.2 The choice offered by the TTO approach
Source: Adapted from Drummond *et al.* (1997)

It has been used predominantly to value health states for chronic disease, although there are some applications that value change in health for temporary health states associated with acute illness. Most applications to date have been in the USA and other high-income countries although there are a few examples from low- and middle-income countries (Tan-Torres 1996; Mahapatra *et al.* 2002).

The advantage of TTO is that by valuing the number of healthy years equivalent for a given time in a particular health state it manages to include a measure of quantity of life into a measure of quality of life. By doing so this produces a ratio scale, which enables the use of parametric statistics. There is also fairly consistent evidence that respondents find TTO easier to understand than the SG. Finally, health is a lived experience over time and this form of presentation therefore has some resonance with reality.

The disadvantages of TTO include the problem of using time as a denominator. First, it confounds issues of time preference because the years of life that are sacrificed come at the end of a life span and therefore may be valued less, suggesting that TTO values are somewhat inflated. Second, it assumes that respondents' perceptions of time are linear, so that the value of a health state remains the same regardless of how long a health state lasts. Other problems levelled at this approach are that:

- it doesn't account for uncertainty (and therefore does not have the theoretical basis of the SG and is an unreal depiction of choices concerning health);
- it requires an interview and therefore, in practice, can be time-consuming and expensive to administer; and
- whilst there is a natural limit of 1.0 for perfect health, there is only an arbitrarily imposed limit of −1.0 for health states considered worse than death.

The standard gamble

This method asks respondents to make a choice between alternative treatments. One treatment offers a certain outcome for a specified health state scenario I for t years. The other option is a treatment that offers a probability (p) of perfect health for t years and ($1-p$) probability of immediate death. With t equal in both treatments, the probability p is varied until the respondent is indifferent between the choices offered and it is this p that is used to weight health state I. Figure 9.3 illustrates the choices offered by the SG. If, for example, a person was indifferent (i.e. felt both options were of equal value to themselves) between ten years with Schistosomiasis and a 70% probability of perfect health, then the quality weight for schistosomiasis would be a 0.7 chance multiplied by 1.0 (the value for full health) = 0.7.

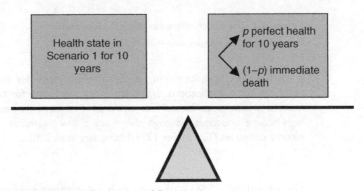

Figure 9.3 The choices offered by the SG method

The SG is based on expected utility theory, as developed by the mathematician John von Neumann and the economist Oscar Morgenstern in the 1940s. According to this theory individuals will rank gambles according to their expected utility (the probability of an event multiplied by the 'value' of an event) and therefore the SG can be used to estimate a cardinal utility function. The theory assumes that individuals act in accordance with particular principles (such as if a person prefers the probability of health state A to B and the probability of health state B to C, then they will also prefer the probability of health state A to C).

The advantages of the SG are that it can produce a cardinal scale and also that it represents choices under uncertainty, which typifies much decision-making in health care. The theory on which it is grounded has also been extensively applied to decision-making in other sectors. In health care, it has been used in several countries to value both chronic and temporary health states. Like TTO, however, it is a time-consuming approach to eliciting preferences and, compared with TTO, respondents often find it a more difficult task to understand (even with the visual aids developed to help picture the choices). The use of probabilities (rather than time) causes two additional difficulties relative to TTO: first, some respondents have an aversion to gambling and are unwilling to choose anything with a risk, which means that values for different health states are equal at zero; second, there are concerns that whilst a gamble approximates some choices made by patients, it does not approximate the choice made in treatment of chronic disease where, for example, treatments for arthritis neither completely cure nor kill patients. Therefore it has been argued that responses can be unreliable and at times invalid.

Descriptions of methods: pre-scored questionnaires (multi-attribute models)

Generating values using the above approaches can be extremely time-consuming. Therefore an alternative is to use pre-scored questionnaires. Examples included the Quality of Well Being Index (QWB), the Health Utilities Index (HUI) and the Euro-Qol Group's EQ-5D. These are based on multi-attribute classifications of health status with each possible health state having an assigned value or utility. The assigned values have been developed amongst a general population using either the VAS, TTO or SG approaches. What this means is that you don't need to run through a valuation exercise each time you want to assess change in utility but instead just ask respondents to complete a multi-attribute health questionnaire. So, how are utility values found using the EQ-5D?

The EQ-5D comprises five dimensions, each with three levels of severity. With two additional states, dead and unconscious, the total number of possible health states is 243 (five dimensions, each at three levels plus the two states dead and unconscious; $3^5 + 2$). There are 21 different value sets from 13 countries (Brooks *et al.* 2003). Outside of Europe, these countries include the USA, Canada, New Zealand, Japan and Zimbabwe. When there is more than one dataset per country, this either reflects use of a different valuation method or collection of values from different parts of a country.

To find the impact on utility from an intervention using a pre-scored questionnaire, it then only becomes necessary to know the health state before and after the intervention to extract the scores and find the difference. Doing this for each patient in a group provides a distribution around a mean difference. Completing the five short questions only take about two minutes and therefore it is very easy to add the EQ-5D to a randomized trial without significantly increasing respondent burden.

Table 9.2 summarizes the approaches to creating index values of health status or HRQL. It also shows that most research began with a national focus and that only one pre-scored questionnaire has been developed with an international focus from the outset: the EQ5D.

Table 9.2 Generic outcome measures available

Geographical focus of original instrument	Approaches to creating index values for health states	
	Scenario-based	Pre-scored questionnaire
National use	TTO	Health Utilities Index (HUI)
	SG	Quality of Well Being Index (QWB)
	Rating scale	15-D
	Ratio scale	SF-6D
	Person trade-off (PTO)	
International use	DALYs (in part)	EQ5D

Combining changes in quantity and quality of life

Combining changes in quantity and quality of life in one index facilitates comparison of a wide set of interventions. There are a number of ways this aggregation might happen. In high-income countries QALYs are the predominant approach and in low- or middle-income countries DALYs are used. Both these methods add successive life years together, given adjustments for quality.

QALYs

Figure 9.4 shows how data on quantity and quality of life is combined using the QALY approach. Without any intervention, assume a person's trajectory of life follows the lower line, with HRQL falling each year until they die (at Death 1). With treatment a person's life follows a different trajectory (the upper line) and HRQL neither falls as rapidly nor does death occur so early. The values of HRQL could correspond, for example, to measurements taken using the EQ-5D over time. The figure shows that treatment leads to gains in HRQL up to point A, after which there is a gain in quantity of life although the HRQL falls each year until death. Total QALYs gained equals the shaded area.

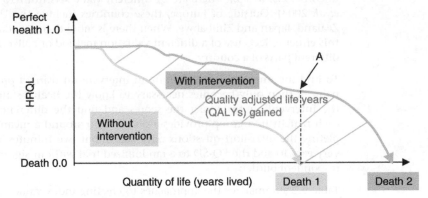

Figure 9.4 QALYs gained from intervention

Source: Adapted from Drummond et al. (1997)

QALYs only combine quantity and quality of life, leaving you to make separate decisions about time preferences and discounting (which you will learn about in Chapter 12). However, there are two other key assumptions implicit in this QALY approach: that each year of life is valued equally across people (i.e. adding a year of full health to a 40-year-old is the same as adding it to a 1-year-old); and that a 10% improvement in health for ten years is equal to adding one year at 100% perfect health.

✏️ **Activity 9.4**

1 Using the ideas presented in Figure 9.4 and the data in Table 9.3, sketch the trajectory of a person's life with and without schistosomiasis and with and without bradycardia (an abnormally slow heartbeat that can sometimes be treated using an implantable pacemaker to control the speed of heartbeats).

Table 9.3 Impact of interventions on quality and quantity of life

Condition	Quality of life index score		Change in quality of life	Quantity of Life		Change in quantity of life
	Before intervention	After intervention		Before intervention	After intervention	
Schistosomiasis	0.3	1.0	0.7	55	56	1
Bradycardia	0.5	1.0	0.5	10	20	10

2 Calculate the QALYs gained from treatment for schistosomiasis and bradycardia.
3 If the total cost of treatment for bradycardia was £20,000 and for schistosomiasis was £50 what would the average cost per QALY gained be?

↻ **Feedback**

1 Your sketches should look something like Figure 9.5.

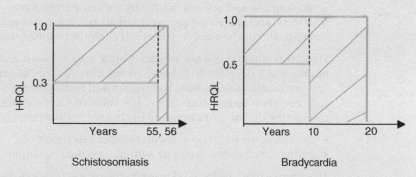

Figure 9.5 Trajectory of person's life before and after treatment for schistosomiasis and bradycardia

2 *Schistosomiasis:* change in quality = 55 × 0.7 = 38.5, change in quantity = 1 × 1.0 = 1.0, Total QALY gain = 39.5. *Bradycardia:* change in quality = 10 × 0.5 = 5, change in quantity = 10 × 0.5 = 5, total QALY gain = 15.

3 *Schistosomiasis:* £50/39.5 = £1.30 per QALY gained. *Bradycardia:* £20,000/15 = £1,333 per QALY gained.

DALYs

DALYs are used to calculate the years of life lost from disease and years lived with a disability for a wide range of diseases and injuries. Both quantity and disability are adjusted for assumptions about age and discounting. Therefore DALYs are one way of measuring the loss from living a shorter life with a disability rather than living a longer life without a disability. DALYs are calculated as weighted combinations of four components, including:

- life expectancy;
- value of life at different ages;
- value of future time; and
- value of avoiding disability.

The value of avoiding disability, to allow comparison with other instruments, will be considered in this chapter. The value and distribution of health at different ages is covered in Chapter 11, and discounting the value of health over time is presented in Chapter 12.

The disability weights behind DALYs are based on descriptions of a condition rather than descriptions of the impact of disease on a person's life or health. Two examples are:

- *blindness*: maximum visual acuity with the best possible correction is less than 3/60 (a person is unable to distinguish the fingers of a hand at 3 metres, or has less than 5% of remaining vision as compared to a normally sighted individual);
- *dementia*: an individual with multiple cognitive deficits that include memory impairment and aphasia (difficulty producing the names of individuals and objects) and apraxia (impaired ability to execute motor activities despite intact motor abilities, sensory function and comprehension of the required task).

These two conditions were weighted on a scale between zero (representing full health) and 1 (representing death), along with 20 other descriptions by 12 international health professionals. They were asked to imagine the social milieu for each state and then to rate and discuss the value of each condition in two ways: by considering the value of extending the lives of healthy people compared with:

- extending the life of people with the specified condition;
- curing the disability of people with the specified condition.

This approach to valuation is known as the person trade-off, and an example of the questions is given in Table 9.4. It has been argued that this approach reflects social decision-making better as the implication of a respondent's choice is clearer (i.e. that one group of patients would not receive care). However uncomfortable this may feel, it is the implicit effect of any future allocation of resources.

Once the 12 experts had provided their values, the median view was the weight adopted for the condition. An arbitrary cutting of the 0–1 scale into seven unequal sizes was used to group the 22 conditions and then to place several hundred other diseases into each category (for which each was assigned the mid-point value of the category). To move from these disability weights for a disease involved multiplying the weight by the proportion of incident cases (although sometimes the steps were estimated together by the same raters). These severity weights were presented for

Table 9.4 The person trade-off exercise used to elicit disability weights for DALYs

Thought experiment 1

You are a decision-maker who has only enough money to buy one of two mutually exclusive health care interventions.

Either **choose Intervention A which will:**

Extend the life of 1000 healthy individuals for exactly one year, at which point they will all die. If you do not purchase this, they will all die today.

Or **choose Intervention B which will:**

Extend the life of n ($\geq$ 1000) *blind* individuals for one year. If you do not purchase this, they will all die today.

Thought experiment 2

You are a decision-maker that has only enough money to buy one of two mutually exclusive health care interventions.

Either **choose Intervention A which will:**

Extend the life of 1000 healthy individuals for exactly one year, at which point they will all die. If you do not purchase this, they will all die today.

Or **choose Intervention B which will:**

Cure the disability of n *blind* individuals, who will live exactly one year with or without the intervention.

With the intervention they will live in perfect health, without the intervention they will continue to live for one year with the given disabling condition.

Source: Fox-Rushby (2002)

use as globally relevant utility weights for adjusted survival data in the construction of DALYs (Murray and Lopez 1996).

DALYs are a tool that uses secondary data (and 'expert' estimates) rather than a tool developed for primary data collection. At present, there is just a list of estimated numbers for health state values for treated and untreated states (without specifying the type of treatment). The values given for each disease state are listed in Murray and Lopez (1996). Since 1996, diseases and conditions have been defined in terms of six dimensions with five levels of severity and a number of community and convenience samples across the world have provided valuations for diseases states (Mahapatra *et al.* 2002), although many of the methods and findings have yet to be published.

 Activity 9.5

1 Where might you look for utility values for a health state, such as blindness?
2 Searching for utility values for blindness would provide values from different countries and population groups, ranging roughly between 0.25–0.7. How might you use the utility scores?
3 If no values existed for the health state you were interested in, what else might you consider doing in a short amount of time? You should consider what you have learnt about existing techniques in this chapter.

Feedback

1 You could conduct a search on the internet for relevant databases or literature; search for and examine published data; or use a valuation formula developed by a health state utility instrument.

2 You could select a mid-point value for a decision model (or a value using your preferred instrument or country) and use the ranges within a sensitivity analysis.

3 You could develop a scenario using best available evidence and ask a group of experts to value the state using existing instruments. Alternatively, a group of patients could complete a valuation instrument like the EQ5D or HUI, and the relevant scoring algorithms used.

Figure 9.6 exemplifies the broad relationship between QALYs and DALYs and that DALYs averted equal QALYs gained. However, to be exactly the same, the quality weights would need to measure the same concepts using the same valuation approaches.

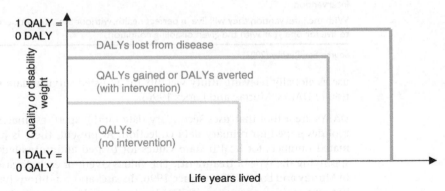

Figure 9.6 Relationship between QALYs and DALYs
Source: Fox-Rushby (2002)

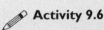
Activity 9.6

Imagine researchers in Brazil were planning to model the cost-utility of screening for and treating tuberculosis among patients with HIV versus doing nothing and they had an opportunity to collect data alongside a randomized trial. Read the excerpt below on the comparative merits of DALYs and EQ5D-based QALYs by Fox-Rushby (2002) and make notes on the issues you would consider prior to advising them whether to use EQ5D-QALYs or DALYs.

  Are DALYs more widely applicable than EQ5D QALYs?

DALYs have been applied more widely and more consistently across more countries and diseases that EQ5D QALYs because the original developers have made the estimates.

However, when DALYs are used by others there are many differences in the inclusion of weights for age and future time as well as different disability weights or even use of the standard expected years of life lost – and yet they are still called DALYs! The EQ5D QALYs have been used more widely in assessing the effectiveness and efficiency of health interventions because this tool has been operationalised for primary data collection e.g. in clinical trials, whereas DALYs have not.

Neither of these instruments evolved from studying conceptions of health in the countries targeted for their use but instead are based on the values of the researchers who developed the instruments, with the EQ5D developers having a wider range of disciplines and countries represented. Therefore neither is likely to represent a universally held view of health, and the 'centre' of the instruments are more likely to represent views held by well-educated, wealthy, white middle-class professionals from Europe and North America.

Are DALYs better than EQ5D QALYs as an outcome measure in economic evaluation?

Evidence on the validity, reliability and sensitivity of the EQ5D is considerable and shows the instrument reaches acceptable standards. However, there is almost no published evidence for DALYs and, coupled with a lack of openness in the design, [this] means there is a significant problem in researchers viewing this as an acceptable measure. EQ5D QALYs are more inclusive than DALYs because they can: include the impact of side-effects; account for the impact of co-morbidities; involve the patient in measuring their own health state; and reflect the values of the general public in particular countries rather than small groups of 'experts'. These criticisms could change only if the DALY was operationalised for use as a primary data collection tool and tested, moved from its concentration on disease to health and improved the reporting of methods and results.

In countries where the EQ5D has not been tested or is not considered relevant, the DALY may be the only option available and therefore used. However, the reliability and validity of the outcome measure must still be questioned (particularly as the disability weights have not been evaluated for any intervention and are unable to distinguish between alternative interventions) and the results subjected to more rigorous sensitivity analysis than is happening currently.

As DALYs and QALYs share the same basic idea of combining the impact of mortality and morbidity into one measure designed for resource allocation, they also share (and are unlikely to shed) some of the same criticisms e.g. discrimination against the aged, and those less likely to return to full health such as the permanently disabled and the poor, and that 'health' rather a broader notion of human welfare is used to allocate resources.

DALYs or QALYs for decision-making?

. . . Cost-effectiveness analysis can be used by decision-makers at several levels, each of which lead to different conclusions about the current relevance of using QALYs relative to DALYs.

International decision-making: DALYs offer a quick broad-brush approach to estimating the impact of interventions for different diseases in different regions of the world based on expert views. [They are] therefore of more interest to international decision-making agencies such as the WHO and World Bank who recommend health policy or allocate loans across countries. QALYs have never been used in this context so provide no data, however rough.

National decision-making: In high-income countries, DALYs offer no advantages over the existing QALY measures. In middle-income countries where there is some development in QALY research, either might be relevant. In low-income countries, where the World Bank ties loans to the calculation of DALYs and where little research income exists for the development of nationally applicable measures, it is unlikely that locally relevant QALYs will be developed for decision-making.

 Feedback

Factors to consider would include: how widely used both measures are in Brazil; the likely use of results and provision of funds for treatment by national and international decision-makers; and the availability of a translated version of the EQ5D in Brazilian Portuguese as well as testing for reliability and validity within the new context. You might also advise them to run a decision model in advance with the best evidence available to judge whether the utility values are likely to influence results (using values from the literature).

What affects utility values for health states?

So far you have learnt about techniques designed to elicit values for different health states. Since undertaking these exercises, researchers have shown that not only do health state values vary by health state but that utility values vary among respondents for the same health state (Allotey *et al.* 2003). Some of the reasons health states vary for the same health state are due to:

- Presentation and use of information:
  - labelling of health states (e.g. giving a name to a disease, presenting information in terms of what can be done rather than what can't be done)
  - willingness to use the whole of the scales available.
- Attitudes of the respondent:
  - willingness to accept risk
  - perception of personal risk
  - time preference.
- Characteristics of respondent:
  - socioeconomic variables
  - demographic profile.
- Personal experience of health and illness:
  - in self or family
  - as a professional.
- Cultural and environmental setting

 Activity 9.7

Why might a rural population in Cameroon weight paraplegia differently from a group of Australian athletes competing in the Paralympics?

Feedback

There are many reasons including: the impact of experience is different due to the underlying level of health and social services (e.g. the provision of bathing aids in a house versus having only a pit latrine away from the home); and, sociodemographic and economic characteristics are likely to be different. You may have suggested other reasons too.

Summary

You have seen how utility scores for health states allow the effects of mortality and the impact of morbidity to be combined into a single comprehensive index and compared across a wide range of interventions and for different diseases. The methods developed allow preferences to be elicited from hypothetical and actual situations, therefore allowing the preferences of patients, professionals and the general public to influence decision-making. Unfortunately, eliciting values is often labour intensive, needs skilled interviewers and respondents can find the tasks difficult to understand.

References

Allotey P, Reidpath D, Kouame A and Cummins R (2003) The DALY, context and the determinants of the severity of disease: an exploratory comparison of paraplegia in Australia and Cameroon. *Social Science and Medicine* 57(5):949–58.

Brooks R, Rabin R and de Charro F (eds) (2003) *The measurement and valuation of health status using the EQ-5D: European perspective* (Evidence from the EuroQol BIOMED research program). Dordrecht: Kluwer Academic Publishers, see also www.euroqol.org/ for updated information.

Drummond MF, O'Brien B, Stoddart GL and Torrance GW (1997) *Methods for the economic evaluation of health care programmes.* Oxford: Oxford Medical Publications.

Fox-Rushby J (2002) *Disability-adjusted life years (DALYs) for decision-making?* London: Office of Health Economics, www.ohe.org/.

Mahapatra P, Salomon JA and Nanda L (2002) Measuring health state values in developing countries – results from a community survey in Andhra Pradesh, in CJL Murray *et al.* (eds) *Summary measures of population health: concepts, ethics, measurement and applications.* Geneva: WHO, pp. 473–85.

Murray CJL and Lopez AD (eds) (1996) *The global burden of disease.* Cambridge, MA: Harvard University Press.

Tan-Torres T (1996) Comparison of different methods of eliciting utilities for outcome states in leprosy. *Journal of Clinical Epidemiology* 49(1):17.

Further reading

Fox-Rushby J and Hanson K (2001) Calculating and presenting disability adjusted life years (DALYs) in cost-effectiveness analysis. *Health Policy and Planning* 16(3):326–31.

Goldstein MK and Tsevat J (n.d.) *Assessing desirability of health outcomes for medical decision-making and cost-effectiveness analysis* (part of series of interactive learning tools), http://symptomresearch.nih.gov/chapter_24/index.htm.

Stalmeier P *et al.* (2001) What should be reported in a methods section on utility assessment? *Medical Decision Making* 21(3):200–7.

Szende A, Schramm W, Flood E, Larson P, Gorina E, Rentz AM and Snyder L (2003) Health-related quality of life assessment in adult haemophilia patients: a systematic review and evaluation of instruments. *Haemophilia* 9(6):678–87.

10 Monetary valuation of health and non-health consequences

Overview

In this chapter you will learn why improvements in health are a necessary but not sufficient indicator of the economic benefits from health care interventions. Two types of economic evaluation that can account for the range of benefits (cost-consequence analysis and cost-benefit analysis) are compared and contrasted. Three broad approaches to valuing benefits in money terms are outlined with some detail of how each can be operationalised.

Learning objectives

After working through this chapter, you will be able to:

- explain why valuing improvements in health utility does not fully capture the economic benefits of health care interventions
- list a range of potential economic benefits of health care interventions
- understand the advantages and disadvantages of measuring but not valuing a full range of benefits for economic analysis
- describe three approaches for valuing health and non-health benefits

Key terms

Compensating variation The maximum a person is willing to pay (accept) to receive a benefit (loss) and keep at the same initial level of utility.

Consumer surplus The difference between what a consumer pays for a good and the maximum they would be willing to pay for it.

Contingent valuation Survey approach to asking individuals to imagine markets exist and to give their willingness to pay (accept) for benefits (losses).

Discrete choice experiment A quantitative market research tool used to model and predict consumers' purchase decisions.

Equivalent variation Willingness to pay (accept) rather than suffer a loss (lose a benefit) and yet be as well off after the change.

Externalities Costs or benefits arising from an individual's production or consumption decision which indirectly affects the well-being of others.

Marginal productivity of labour The extra output produced by each additional unit of labour.

Public good A good or service that can be consumed simultaneously by everyone and from which no one can be excluded.

Introduction

If individuals are willing to give up something in order to receive a new good or service, then the new good or service has an opportunity cost and therefore a value. Valuing health state utilities allows the impact of interventions on quantity and quality of life to be measured and valued by trading off these types of benefits against each other.

Unfortunately, health utility indices may not capture the full value of health interventions if the underlying descriptive and therefore measurement system is crude. They can be insensitive to smaller changes in health and therefore imply that small changes, even if they occur across an entire population, have no value. This is a common complaint of the EQ5D and people argue that if only the change were measurable, then it would be valued. Second, the measures focus only on final health outcomes when people may also place value on the processes of the care. Finally, no aspects of human welfare other than health, such as the benefits of children attending more schooling or the impact on family income, are valued directly. If a government wants to maximize welfare from public investment rather than health gain, then this is a particularly strong criticism of using only QALY-type measures to assess the benefits of health care interventions.

In this chapter you will learn about the range of utility-generating aspects of health care interventions and the extent to which different methods of valuing benefits in terms of money can provide a more inclusive measure of value.

What other aspects of utility should also be measured?

Moving away from health utility indices raises the question of what other aspects of utility should be measured, followed closely by the question 'and how?'

Listed below are additional benefits that might arise from health care interventions that are not measured using health indices:

- satisfaction with services (e.g. spending longer with a health care professional or receiving more accurate or quicker results from screening tests);
- small health changes (e.g. less breathlessness when walking);
- changes in income (e.g. directly through impact on work or indirectly through improved education);
- value of information (e.g. results from tests);
- value of feeling cared for, even if no health benefits exist;
- side-effects and fear of them;
- protection from financial risk – particularly catastrophic risk that sends an entire family into poverty;
- change in current and future access to care (e.g. setting up new community clinics);
- institutional and capacity development that increase the abilities of individuals or institutions to lead or adapt more easily to change;
- non-health outcomes (e.g. delivery of new services may raise the profile of a community in the eyes of government officials, leading to provision of other services or more opportunities for trade).

Health status indices have all concentrated on asking individuals about the benefits of interventions to themselves. However, some interventions (e.g. information provided freely on the internet) have public good characteristics and therefore it is not possible to stop people consuming that information. Eliciting values for such goods suffers from a 'free rider' problem as people undervalue their benefits in the belief that others would provide the good and then could not stop use. Alternatively, other interventions have externalities so that consumption has either positive or negative effects on another person. For example, the benefits of impregnated bed nets that kill mosquitoes not only affect those sleeping under the net but also those sleeping near the net. Both these cases show that value can be conferred beyond the individual. It is also the case that individuals may place some value on keeping some services available, so they have an option to use them in the future in case they need to. People may also simply care that services are available for other people even if they do not need or benefit from them directly or indirectly themselves. None of these values are currently included within QALY calculations.

How should the full range of benefits be measured and valued?

When working outside of cost-effectiveness, cost-utility and cost-minimization analysis, the two options are cost-consequence analysis (CCA) and cost-benefit analysis (CBA). The first of these simply presents a listing of costs and consequences of interventions to decision-makers. As Coast (2004) argues, this allows decision-makers to see what is included and how, rather than having to use indices that are based on assumptions they may not understand or adhere to. It also allows decision-makers to put their own values on each cost and consequence and for decision-makers in different settings to place different values on the same set of costs and consequences. A cost-consequence approach is a good way to specify the identification and measurement of benefits and presents a useful opportunity to consider how benefits might be valued in monetary terms. However, decision-makers' values may not match those of the public or patients and the values used may also become inscrutable.

Considering the value of opportunities foregone should be the basis for valuing benefits and it can help avoid having to impose your values onto other people. In the last chapter, for example, the TTO focused on giving up time lived in the future to gain healthy time now. In this chapter you will consider money.

Money represents a claim on consumption so loss of money can represent the value of things lost (and vice versa). The advantage of using money is that people are used to it (although to different degrees) and used to making their own decisions with it. It is the unit of exchange for goods and services and can therefore be used to value and add up many different benefits. It also provides a common unit for comparing against costs. Using monetary values moves evaluation into the realms of CBA. Its base in welfare economics considers individuals to be the best judge of their welfare and therefore the focus is on what choices individuals make.

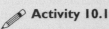 **Activity 10.1**

Look at Table 10.1 which shows how the characteristics of two treatments for the same disease differ.

Table 10.1 Comparison of two treatments for the same disease

	Treatment A	Treatment B
Cost of intervention to health service	£30	£1000
Annual probability of need	0.002	0.002
Mortality	3%	3%
Mean (SD) score on functional ability*	0.65 (0.23)	0.82 (0.1)
Mean (SD) number of nights sleep disturbed per month	15 (5.2)	25 (4.3)
Patient satisfaction		Compared with Treatment B, those with Treatment A are significantly more satisfied with speed of service and confidence in staff, wide confidence intervals elsewhere
Mean (SD) score for carer quality of life*	0.85 (0.2)	0.7 (0.3)
Rate of severe adverse reaction	0.06%	0.1%
Mean (SD) time unable to work	21 days (10)	40 days (30)
Availability per 1 million head of population	20 000	500 000

* A higher score is better

1 Which treatment would you prefer to adopt and why?
2 If you knew that Treatment A was care in a primary health centre and Treatment B was care in a district hospital would you want to know about any other benefits or costs?
3 How else might you consider valuing this range of benefits?

 Feedback

1 There is no correct answer here, it will reflect your opinion. You should be aware of which types of information you placed more weight on and consider whether you ignored any information as unimportant.

2 You may want to know about: costs falling on patients and others, such as transport to hospital; whether this is an infectious disease and therefore the impact of treatment on transmission rates; the impact on provision of other services within each type of setting; and the satisfaction of service providers. You may have considered other factors as well.

3 One or more of the benefits could be combined into one scenario and respondents asked to value the state using the TTO or SG. Alternatively a monetary approach might be used. As there is no change in mortality or annual probability of need, these might be excluded.

Methods of monetary valuation

Being aware of Oscar Wilde's view of a cynic (*a man who knows the price of everything but the value of nothing*), the approaches you will learn about will indeed acknowledge that some prices do not reflect value and therefore should not be used for valuing the benefits of interventions. However, some approaches are, at least theoretically, able to reflect value.

Table 10.2 shows three main approaches used to value benefits of health care interventions in terms of money: human capital theory; observed preferences; and stated preferences.

Table 10.2 Approaches used to value benefits in money terms

Approach	Example
Human capital theory	View body as a productive machine for the economy and value time out of paid work
Observed preferences 1 Decision makers a) implicit public sector values b) court awards	 a) investment in road safety/number of lives saved b) sum paid through court case won for an injury (rough guidelines available)
2 Individuals a) wage-risk trade-off b) expenditure on insurance c) purchase of risk-reducing goods	 a) multiplication of premium paid for risky jobs by change in risk faced (e.g. steeplejacks) b) sum for which lives or limbs are insured c) cost or product multiplied by change in risks faced (e.g. smoke alarm)
Stated preferences a) Contingent valuation	 a) stated sums people would be willing to pay to accept a reduction in risk of changing quality or quantity of life, contingent on a market existing (e.g. WTP for % chance of being free of cardiac symptoms or for clean air)
b) Discrete choice experiment	b) An attitude-based survey measure of value designed to assess the value of attributes contributing to overall value

Human capital theory

Human capital theory views the role of individuals rather like that of a machine, as their contribution to gross national product. When wages equal the marginal product of labour, an appropriate indicator of value is the wage paid. Therefore, many early CBAs estimated the value gained from investing in health (by individuals or the state) as expected change in earnings. For example, for a change in quantity of life multiply the reduction (or gain) in life years by expected earnings for the remainder of that life or for a change in health multiply any reduction (or gain) in productivity by change in earnings.

This approach is rooted in an accepted conception of health, where people are viewed in terms of activities or bodily functioning. Indeed, expressions used to describe fit bodies can liken them to a well-oiled machine. The advantages of this approach are that the empirical valuation of life becomes a well-defined problem requiring only a set of mortality tables and individuals earnings to calculate benefits and that it indicates the health programmes which have a high impact on national income.

There are many problems with using the human capital approach. First is the major concern that value is only measured in terms of productivity, denying any consumption value. Second, labour markets may not exist (e.g. for the elderly or children) or may not be functioning freely, which means there may be no market price, or that market prices reflect things other than productivity (e.g. the extent of unionization, discrimination, level of unemployment). Using existing market values within economic evaluation may direct care away from the very young, unemployed and others. Third, estimating how productivity is affected by health status is complex not only because of the two-way relationship (who works is determined by health and more productive people may also spend more maintaining health) but also because health tends to be measured in a simplistic way in such studies (e.g. cases of malaria, number of days ill, body mass index or activities of daily living).

Observed preferences

Observing the choices that people make in practice can be a good indicator of value as people make decisions in real situations rather than in hypothetical experiments. Table 10.2 shows this can rely on decision-makers' or an individual's values. The problem is that real situations are complex and the results can't always be taken as an indicator of value for another situation. For example, many court cases may be settled out of court for undisclosed sums so awards are a biased reflection of all values. In addition, the sums awarded may be based on earnings potential and reflect not only compensation for injury but punishment for a defendant's breach in duty of care.

There are some situations in which individuals can be observed trading-off risk of death and injury for increased wealth (e.g. higher salaries for window cleaners of tall buildings) or paying for goods that reduce the risk (e.g. smoke detectors, safer airlines). The willingness to accept (WTA) money for a higher risk or the willingness to pay (WTP) to reduce risk can be used to estimate an implied value of life.

Activity 10.2

Airline A	1/100,000 mortality rate	£395 return ticket London–Nairobi
Airline B	1/130,000 ” ”	£430 ” ” ” ”

1 What is the implied value of life for a person choosing to fly with Airline B?
2 If a researcher observed your purchase of airline tickets and valued your life and health in this way, what objections could you raise?

Feedback

1 Implied value of life = (£430 − £395) × (130,000 − 100,000) = £1,050,000.

2 You may not know the actual risks or you may perceive the risks to be different; the prices offered can change over time but risks stay the same; and you only pay one price but there may be several different risks (to health and life) and it is not possible to separate out the impacts. You may think of other objections too.

Stated preferences

Table 10.2 showed two methods for eliciting stated preferences: contingent valuation and discrete choice experiments. Both methods ask individuals to make judgements in a hypothetical situation. Contingent valuation asks people directly about their maximum willingness to pay for a good or service contingent on a market existing. Discrete choice experiments present two (or more) scenarios to a person and ask them to choose which one they prefer. Each scenario describes a number of attributes about the option, with each option differing in the levels of each attribute. When the scenarios include a cost attribute within the choice, WTP can be estimated.

Valuations using stated preference techniques with WTP are rooted in consumer surplus and capture the difference between the amount a consumer is willing to pay for a good and the amount actually paid. Increments of consumer surplus are equated with increases in consumer welfare. As you know that consumption confers utility to a consumer, you accept that money confers utility indirectly as it represents a claim on consumption. Therefore you can state that any increase in WTP represents more utility to the consumer.

Two methods can be used to measure consumer surplus: compensating or equivalent variations, both of which can be divided into WTP and WTA. The most common approach is to ask an individual for their WTP for a new intervention using the compensating variation approach. This would value the maximum a person was willing to pay for a benefit (e.g. reduction in risk of death, or increased likelihood of better health).

There is some concern about income and double counting benefits when asking about WTP. For example, if a person considers a health gain may increase their income, they may increase their stated WTP. Not clarifying whether or not respondents should account for any change in income may mean that respondents do not consider this consistently and thus there may be a biased explanation of variation in WTP

Contingent valuation questionnaires and scenarios need to be designed with care. There are many aspects to consider including:

* developing the scenario;
* payment and response options;
* how best to convey any risks simply and accurately;
* the time period to consider for the scenario and payment;
* usual aspects related to good survey design.

Once WTP values have been elicited, the total gain in welfare needs to be calculated. The simplest approach is to add up the WTP across individuals affected by the programme (i.e. gainers willing to pay > 0 or losers willing to accept < 0 for the policy) and across time.

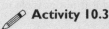

Activity 10.3

Table 10.3 summarizes the values from a contingent valuation exercise.

Table 10.3 Values from a contingent valuation exercise

Individual	WTP (+) or WTA (−)	
	Intervention 1	Intervention 2
1	+130	+12
2	−20	+44
3	+10	−65
4	+55	−23
5	−25	+24
6	+80	+89
7	+63	+79
8	−18	+23
9	+43	+55
10	−2	−10

WTP = willingness to pay
WTA = willingness to accept

Using the values:

1 What intervention has the greatest welfare gain?
2 How much do the gainers have to compensate the losers in Intervention 1 and 2?
3 Assume that this compensation is not actually paid and that those who lose out from the interventions are the poorest people. Why might you want to account for this and how?
4 What problem could you foresee in studies that only ask questions about WTP? You need to think about a programme which causes problems for some people.

Feedback

1 You need to add up the figures in each column under Intervention 1 and 2. Intervention 1 has a higher welfare gain, with a total of £316 compared with £228 for intervention 2.

2 You need to sum the value of negative values. £65 and £98 are needed to compensate losers for interventions 1 and 2 respectively.

3 WTP is constrained by income, so those with higher incomes tend to be willing to pay more for the same health impact. The relative size of income of those losing and gaining could be compared and an adjustment made. You will learn about various approaches in the next chapter.

4 There is no possibility for people to pay less than zero in a WTP study. Therefore there may be many zero values that are not 'true' zeros because they don't reflect negative values. Not including negative values is therefore likely to lead to an over-estimation of benefit as those who lose out from a project don't get to indicate how strongly they lose out as their views are not captured by a minimum WTA question One of the reasons researchers often don't include WTA questions is that responses don't always reflect these 'negative values' and, as they are unconstrained by income, respondents can give enormous numbers that dominate the analysis and yet don't reflect minimum WTA values in practice.

Discrete choice experiments can also provide values for entire scenarios. In a discrete choice experiment, individuals are presented with two choices and asked which choice they would make. Within one experiment, each respondent would be offered several choices. Each choice would have the same attributes (eg cost, who delivers the service, type of test, discomfort of procedure) but the levels on each would vary (e.g. cost for Clinic A might be £10, £35 or £75 depending on the levels set in advance of the experiment and the service might be provided by either a GP, nurse or utility specialist). The value of each attribute is estimated using regression analysis. The construction of attributes and levels might be selected during qualitative research among patients and providers and selection of the mix through techniques of experimental design. The complexity in experimental design means that discrete choice experiments are only worthwhile if the aim is to establish the trade-offs people are willing to make for different attributes of the intervention offered rather than just establish WTP for the intervention as a whole.

There are many advantages of using stated preferences:

- individuals are asked about explicit changes in risks directly so responses don't have to be inferred, which allows analysis of explicit preferences and utility;
- they can be applied to any situation and not limited to existing market situations;
- the relationship between individual WTP for risk reduction and other factors like initial risk level, size of risk reduction, income and age can be investigated directly;
- because money is the denominator, the utility function is broader than just HRQ;
- contingent valuation and choice experiments (with WTP) can be used to estimate welfare change.

There are a number of challenges faced when using stated preference techniques. First, the theoretical base is questioned as consumers may not always be considered to be the best judges of their own welfare. Second, the technique is open to bias because respondents can find the hypothetical situation difficult to understand or deliberately shape their answers to facilitate an outcome. Alternatively, researchers can mis-specify the scenario, payment options or analysis. Finally there are many practical problems such as having low response rates to surveys, deciding how much of what information to give in a scenario and determining who is the appropriate respondent (e.g. current or future patients). As a result many studies currently suffer from using small non-random samples.

Summary

You have learnt about the need to consider a wide range of benefits that might arise from a health care intervention. You went on to consider three ways of determining the monetary value of the benefits of an intervention: human capital theory; observed preferences; and stated preferences. You will now go on to consider issues of equity in the valuation of outcomes.

References

Coast J (2004) Is economic evaluation in touch with society's health values? *British Medical Journal* 329:1233–6, http://bmj.bmjjournals.com/cgi/content/extract/329/7476/1233.

Further reading

Bateman IJ *et al.* (2002) *Economic valuation with stated preferences techniques: a manual.* Cheltenham: Edward Elgar Publishing.
Bhatia M and Fox-Rushby J (2002) Willingness to pay for treated mosquito nets in Surat, India: the design and descriptive analysis of a household survey. *Health Policy and Planning* 17(4): 402–11.
Schultz TP (2004) Health economics and applications in developing countries. *Journal of Health Economics* 23(4):637–41.
Smith RD (2003) Construction of the contingent valuation market in health care: a critical assessment. *Health Economics* 12(8):609–28.

Issues concerning equity in the valuation of outcomes

Overview

In the previous chapters you learnt about approaches to measure and value health or welfare. They all assumed that maximization of health or welfare was the ultimate desire of a society. However, people may have preferences for how health and welfare should be distributed. If so, then any valuation should account for preferences about this distribution and this may mean that people are willing to sacrifice some gains in health or welfare for a different distribution. In this chapter you will learn about a technical approach to considering whether people have a preference for the distribution of benefits within a population and whether there are any distributional implications within existing health state valuation techniques.

Learning objectives

After working through this chapter, you will be able to:

- explain why equity weights might be needed in addition to counting QALYs or other benefits
- explain how existing health state valuation techniques have distributional implications embedded in responses
- debate the case for and against age-weights

Key terms

Diminishing marginal utility (of income or life years) Each additional monetary unit or each additional year of life gives a little less satisfaction than the last.

Social welfare function This describes the preferences of an individual over social states. It is accepted to be a function of equity and efficiency.

Introduction

In the last few chapters you have looked at alternative ways of measuring and valuing gains in the capacity to benefit (either in terms of health or welfare). Little has been said about whether people have preferences for the way that benefits are distributed among the population or whether the valuation techniques used could have any impact on the distribution of resources.

In this chapter you will see how valuation techniques can force respondents into adopting particular views on how resources should be distributed and provide results that have in-built implications for the distribution of resources. The chapter ends with some evidence of how strongly people feel about the distribution of benefits and how values concerning distribution might be built into the design and interpretation of economic evaluations.

Do people have preferences about the distribution of health interventions?

✎ Activity 11.1

The concept of a 'social welfare function' links the size of welfare gain with the distribution of gain. Figure 11.1 shows the trade-off between size and distribution of welfare gain, which is reflected as an 'indifference curve'. An indifference curve is the combinations of two goods (or services or characteristics) that leave the consumer with the same level of utility.

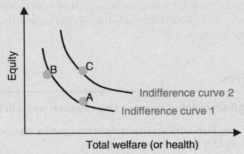

Figure 11.1 Trade-off between size and distribution of welfare gain
Source: LSHTM

1 Rank the interventions A to C in order of preference.
2 On the graph, sketch the size of gain in health or wealth that society is willing to lose in order to achieve more equity by moving from Intervention A to Intervention B.
3 Think of an example for Interventions A, B and C.

↻ Feedback

1 C = 1 (most preferred), A = 2.5 and B = 2.5 (middle of tied ranks as equally preferred).

2 The size of loss of total welfare is the difference between A and B on the horizontal axis.

3 Given a fixed budget for a new vaccination, two positions could be selected: providing as many new vaccinations as possible, which would mean focusing on high-density populations or choosing to go to all geographical areas equally and therefore vaccinate fewer people in the urban areas; or an increase in the budget would allow more of both to be achieved (and hence move to position C).

The ratio of health or welfare effects for Intervention A and B per head of population in Figure 11.1 would define the size of preference to avoid inequitable distribution of benefits.

Lindholm *et al.* (1998) asked 631 elected citizens in Sweden to compare the size and distribution of benefits of different health care interventions. They were given information about deaths amongst blue- and white-collar workers before and after different interventions and were asked to choose which intervention they preferred (assuming all costs were the same). They found that 58% of politicians preferred losing ten lives to achieve greater equity but that as the 'cost' of achieving equity rose (i.e. cost more lives) the percentage decreased. If resource allocation is to reflect the views of politicians, it should not be restricted to health maximization but also account for who receives the benefits.

Whilst preferences for the trade-off between the size and distribution of health gain might vary among different groups within a country as well as across countries, it does indicate that a trade-off might exist. Given this possibility, it is important to examine the implications of using health state valuation techniques.

The distributional implications of approaches used to value changes in health and welfare

One of the most common concerns with using WTP to value benefits is that values are positively related to income. This can be seen in Figure 11.2 where income (Y) varies on the x-axis and the utility of health (H) and Y vary on the y-axis. Even though there is a diminishing marginal utility of income (seen by the decreasing slope of $U(H_0Y)$), the person at the higher income level (Y_a) gives a higher utility value to the same health state H_0 than does the person at the lower income level (Y_b).

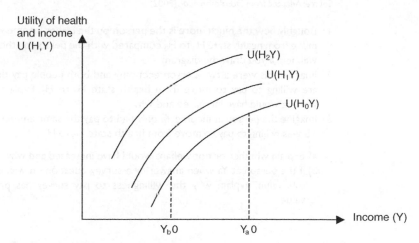

Figure 11.2 Willingness and ability to pay (1)

Source: Adapted from Donaldson *et al.* (2002)

Would richer people be willing to pay more for a change in health state from H_0 to H_1? Figure 11.3 shows that a person on income Y_a0 would be willing to reduce their income to Y_a1 to move from health state H_0 to H_1 *whilst keeping their utility constant.* The person on the lower income would be willing to give up Y_b0 to Y_b1 of their income to move from health state H_0 to H_1 *whilst keeping their utility constant.*

Activity 11.2

Looking at Figure 11.3:

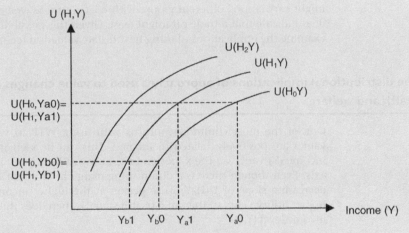

Figure 11.3 Willingness and ability to pay (2)
Source: Adapted from Donaldson *et al.* (2002)

1   Roughly how the much more is the person on the higher income willing to pay in to move from health state H_0 to H_2 compared with the person on the lower income? It will help if you draw the diagram.
2   Imagine this were a two-person economy and both people pay the maximum they are willing to pay to move from health state H_0 to H_2. Explain whether or not welfare would have increased and why.
3   Imagine the person at income Ya only had to pay the same amount as the person at Yb was willing to pay to move from health state H_0 to H_2:

   a) explain whether or not welfare would have increased and why
   b) if the person at Ya when answering a survey question on willingness to pay gave this value, explain why the willingness to pay survey has produced a biased value.

Feedback

1   The amount the person with the higher income (person 'a' at Y_a0) is willing to pay is roughly 50% more than the person on the lower income. Compare the distances in brackets on the x-axis in Figure 11.4 and you will see WTPa > WTPb.

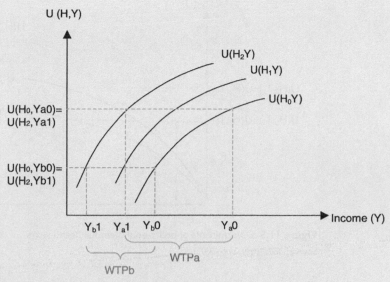

Figure 11.4 Willingness and ability to pay (3)

Source: Adapted from Donaldson *et al.* (2002)

2 There would be no overall change in welfare because this change in income (e.g. Y_b0 to Y_b1) keeps utility constant at (i.e. $U(H_0, Y_b0) = U(H_2, Y_b1)$). Notice the maximum a person is WTP is the horizontal distance.

3 a) Welfare would increase because person a is able to gain an increase in health and keep some of the income they would have been willing to pay. Therefore person a can spend the money on something else and increase their utility.

   b) WTP survey questions should always ask for a person's *maximum* WTP because this implies utility will be kept constant. A maximum WTP is the point at which a person is indifferent between a reduction in their income and an improvement in their health, so the welfare gain from losing income equals the welfare gain from better health for that person. If a lower value is given, it implies that the full value of the benefit is not reflected and therefore the WTP is biased downwards.

The impact of income on WTP values means that estimates of utility based on WTP accord more value to those with higher incomes. A WTP of £1 therefore does not represent equal value across all people and the use of unadjusted WTP values may change the distribution of welfare in favour of those with higher incomes. Two responses to this knowledge have been to use non-monetary methods of valuation, such as the TTO and SG approaches (covered in Chapter 9), and to find appropriate weights for adjusting WTP values so they are better able to reflect the 'shadow price' (i.e. true social value) for a change in welfare.

There has been little questioning of the distributional implications of non-monetary valuation techniques and many have assumed that the use of life years and QALYs in economic evaluation avoids the distributional problems of CBA. However, Donaldson *et al.* (2002) have shown that this is not the case.

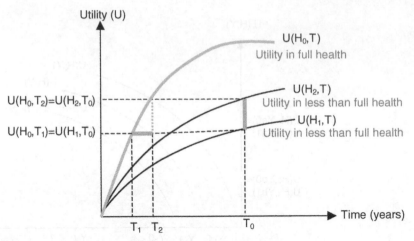

Figure 11.5 Determinants of utility-equivalent full health years
Source: Donaldson *et al.* (2002)

Figure 11.5 shows a curve representing the utility of full health $U(H_0)$ over successive years (T). Like income, the curve is convex which implies that each additional year of full health is of slightly less value than the previous year. This follows the common finding, and therefore assumption, of diminishing marginal returns to increasing amounts of a good or service. The TTO asks people to consider how many years of full health they are willing to give up for a longer life in a poorer health state. Therefore the TTO seeks to find the number of years in full health that give the same level of utility as the number of years in poorer health. Figure 11.5 shows that improving health by moving from health state H_1 to H_2 is equal in terms of utility to a reduction in years of full health from T_2 to T_1.

 Activity 11.3

In Activity 11.2 and Figure 11.3 the possibility that people had different amounts of money available and the impact this might have on the size of WTP were considered. Consider Figure 11.5 and answer the following questions:

1 How might people answering TTO questions have a different amount of time available?
2 How would you expect this to impact on values given?
3 What implications might this have on interpreting results?

 Feedback

1 People may have different life expectancies and/or may be 'given' a different length of 'potential life' in studies using TTO to elicit health states valuations.

2 Someone with (or 'given') a longer life expectancy will trade more years for the same health gain than a person with a lower life expectancy. Therefore, younger people are

more likely to have higher utility scores for the same improvements in health states compared with older people (see Figure 11.6).

3 TTO creates an incentive to allocate resources to younger people and to countries with higher life expectancies (on health state utility values alone).

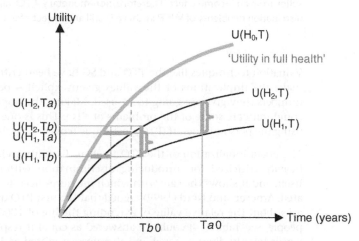

Figure 11.6 Utility equivalents full health years and remaining life expectancy
Source: Donaldson *et al.* (2002)

Figure 11.6 shows two people (*a* & *b*) with different lengths of life ahead of them. With more time available, person *a* is willing to give up more years compared with person *b* for the same change in health state (from H$_1$ to H$_2$) *whilst keeping their own utility constant*. Therefore, because the length of time available cannot be controlled, TTO values that are not adjusted to account for age are likely to be biased. A QALY is unlikely to be of equal value to people with different life expectancies and the use of unadjusted QALYs may change the distribution of welfare in favour of those with greater life expectancy. However, the story of bias does not end here.

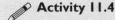 **Activity 11.4**

1 Explain whether or not you think richer or poorer people are likely to have longer lives and why.
2 To what extent do QALYs based on TTO values get round the distribution problems of WTP values?

Feedback

> 1 Richer people (and countries) have a higher life expectancy at birth and through life. This effect may be direct (in being able to access health care when needed) and indirect (through its association with better social conditions). The direction of the relationship is also debated; poverty causing ill health and vice versa.
>
> 2 Because wealth is positively related to life expectancy, TTO values are also likely to suffer from an income effect. Therefore, non-monetary TTO values don't get round the distribution problems of WTP as there is still an indirect effect.

Valuation techniques like the TTO and SG have been criticized because they don't make the implications of the values given explicit – people can't tell how the numbers they give are going to be used. Making the implication of values clearer could mitigate some of the problems of TTO. This is one of the reasons given for using the person trade-off (PTO) technique (covered in Chapter 9).

The operationalization of the PTO to elicit disability weights for DALYs has been heavily criticized for introducing discrimination within the valuation process itself, and it shows the care with which measures need to be developed and evaluated. Arnesen and Nord (1999) argued that the first PTO question of DALYs (which asks about the relative value of extending the life of 1000 sighted and 1000 blind people, see Table 9.4) could be answered as equal if respondents valued disabled versus healthy lives as equal and therefore weighted as 1.0. The second question ('thought experiment') is different and does not require that a final weight of less than 1 be based on a supposition that the lives of disabled people are worth less than those of the able-bodied. If an expert considers that relieving 5000 people of blindness is as valuable as prolonging the lives of 1000 healthy people, the state 'blindness' would be weighted 0.2. Both positions are logical. However, the DALY development process then forced respondents to make their valuations 'consistent', by taking a mean value. This 'forced consistency' means that disability weights from DALYs do not reflect the preferences of respondents and introduces bias by discriminating against the value of disabled lives. In this case the first PTO question could be dropped from the valuation exercise.

Equity weighted outcome measures

Given that people have a preference for the distribution of benefits in a population and that existing valuation techniques have distributional implications themselves, there have been increasing calls to re-weight the values for health and welfare benefits. The aim of using equity weights for QALYs would be to reflect social value as well as health gain. The issues that proceed are threefold: what concepts of equity or justice should be reflected? What variables should be represented? And what specific weight should be used?

QALYs are based on utilitarian principles that seek to maximize the size of health gain or capacity to benefit. However, other theoretical stances that have different distributive implications offer other possibilities. For example, the political philosopher John Rawls would argue for improving the position of those who are worst off in society by increasing their opportunities for access to health gain. Adopting an egalitarian approach might seek to equalize health and an entitlements approach seek to equalize opportunities. In the health field, other approaches to equity have included: the 'rule of rescue', where those lives in imminent danger are saved first; equal access for equal need (and unequal access for unequal need); and the 'fair innings', which aims to eliminate disparities in length of life or QALYs according to expectations of a 'normal' life span. Each philosophy offers different decision-making rules with associated advantages and disadvantages.

There are many variables posited for equity weighting of outcome measures, including age, sex, socioeconomic status, education or ethnicity. Within the health field, most focus has been on varying values by age. For example, DALYs contain an age-weighting factor because it was argued that certain age groups not only contributed more to the production of an economy but also that younger and older people were often dependent on the same middle-aged groups for caring. Therefore it was argued that society should want these age groups to receive more health care.

Four arguments have been used to question the weighting of DALYs by age (Fox-Rushby 2002). First, a principle of 'universalism of life' has been invoked to justify that the value per life year should be common to all people regardless of their age. Second, using notions of dependency discriminates against those with fewer dependencies and social ties. As much of health care is given to an individual rather than on the basis of other people's dependency on them, such principles could be considered irrelevant as an ethical base for allocating health care resources. Third, the premises for weighting DALYs have been used inconsistently. For example, to weight by age because it captures different social roles is not consistent with the decision to ignore a person's occupation or income or productivity. Finally, age weighting may double count values if the value of living a healthy life at different ages is not considered separately from the impact of disability during the valuation process.

As Tsuchiya (1999) wrote, the age-weighting of DALYs is an efficiency weight rather than an equity weight because it is linked to productivity (either at home or work). This contrasts with the egalitarian basis of the 'fair innings' approach that considers past, present and future life (or QALY) expectancy with people of the same age given a different weight depending on their expected lifetime QALYs. As Figure 11.7 shows, this gives a different pattern of weighting by age. In Figure 11.7, social classes I and II would begin with an equity weight of around 1.2 for every QALY gained in the first year of life compared with an equity weight of around 0.8 for those in social classes IV and V. This means that more weight would be given to increasing the life expectancy and health of social classes I and II. This, in turn, would encourage more investment in health care for these social classes relative to QALY measures that weighted gains equally across the social classes.

Questions concerning the evidence basis for age-weights can be considered in the light of Tsuchiya's (1999) review of nine empirical studies conducted in countries with high incomes and long life expectancies. She found limited empirical evidence that people value health benefits differently depending on the age at which a person receives health care but no evidence to support a standard uniform

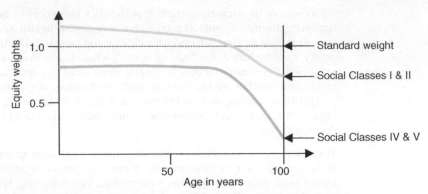

Figure 11.7 Equity weights by the fair innings argument: UK males by social class for a fair innings of 61 QALYs
Source: Tsuchiya (1999)

weighting. There appears to be broad agreement that the profile declines after middle age but some disagreement about whether there is a peak in middle age. These relationships appear to hold regardless of the age of the respondent. However, she concluded that the evidence to suggest a particular rate for efficiency-based age weights is extremely limited and that evidence for equity-based weights was almost non-existent.

Summary

You have seen that people have preference for the distribution of health benefits, and that they are willing to sacrifice health gains in a population for a more equal distribution in health gain. You have also learnt that health state valuation techniques have a built-in bias that favours wealthier members of society – and that this is not limited to monetary valuation techniques like WTP but also applies to non-monetary techniques like the TTO. Therefore there seems to be a twofold justification for using equity-weighted values for changes in QALYs or DALYs. Age-weights for DALYs was used to distinguish efficiency from equity weights and an example of the impact of using social class as an equity weight over different ages was given. However, whilst there is sufficient evidence that equity weights are desired there is a paucity of evidence on appropriate rates.

References

Arnesen T and Nord E (1999) The value of DALY life: problems with ethics and validity of disability adjusted life years. *British Medical Journal* 319(7222): 1423–5.

Donaldson C, Birch S and Gafni A (2002) The distribution problem in economic evaluation: income and the valuation of costs and consequences of health care programmes. *Health Economics* 11(1):55–70.

Fox-Rushby JA (2002) *Disability-adjusted life years (DALYs) for decision-making?* London: Office of Health Economics.

Lindholm L, Rosén M and Emmelin M (1998) How many lives is equity worth? A proposal for equity adjusted years of life saved. *Journal of Epidemiology and Community Health* 52: 808–11.

Tsuchiya (1999) Age-related preferences and age weighting health benefits. *Social Science and Medicine* 48(2):267–76.

Further reading

Sassi F, Archard L and Le Grand J (2001) Equity and the economic evaluation of healthcare. *Health Technology Assessment* 5(3), www.hta.nhsweb.nhs.uk/fullmono/mon503.pdf.

Discounting

Overview

In this chapter you will learn about the challenge of comparing interventions which differ in the timing of their costs and effects. Economists are generally convinced that individuals and societies have a positive rate of time preference – that is, other things being equal, individuals and societies prefer additional consumption now to in the future, and similarly prefer additional consumption in the near future to the distant future. In the case of costs it is assumed that individuals prefer to incur costs later rather than sooner. As a consequence, it is suggested that future costs and effects be discounted and expressed as present values in order to better inform current decision-making.

Learning objectives

After working through this chapter, you will be able to:

- **understand the reasons for discounting**
- **re-express a stream of future costs and benefits as a present value**
- **establish the impact of discounting on decision options**
- **determine when discounting is necessary**

Key terms

Axiom of stationarity The assumption that preference for one intervention over another will be unchanged if both are either brought forward in time or postponed by the same amount.

Catastrophic risk The likelihood that there will be some event so devastating that all returns from a programme or intervention are eliminated, or at least radically and unpredictably altered.

Compounding The process by which savings grow with the payment of interest.

Discount factor The present value expressed as a proportion of the undiscounted value.

Discount rate The rate at which future costs and outcomes are discounted to account for time preference.

Elasticity The percentage change in one variable relative to the percentage change in another.

Intergenerational equity The fair treatment of future generations by preceding generations.

> **Present value** The worth of a future benefit or cost in terms of their value now.
>
> **Pure time preference** An individual's preference for consumption now rather than later, with an unchanging level of consumption per capita over time.

Comparing costs and effects which differ in their timing

It is common for the costs of an intervention to be generated largely in the near future and for its benefits to accrue in the distant future. For example, there may be costs associated with diagnosis and treatment now, and as a consequence the patient lives longer, and enjoys a higher HRQL in the future. How can you tell whether these future benefits justify the increase in current costs? Obviously the size of the benefits relative to the size of the costs will be important. But should you also be concerned about the timing of these benefits? Does it matter how long you have to wait for these benefits?

Different interventions can differ dramatically in the timing of their costs and effects. For some, the costs may largely be upfront, whilst for others they may arise over several years. For some interventions the benefits may be received almost straightaway and for others not start for several years. How can you compare projects with very different time profiles? For example, how can you compare smoking cessation programmes with the treatment of lung cancer? Again the relative magnitudes will be important but how can you take account of differences in timing?

The solution recommended by economists is to re-express the streams of costs and streams of benefits as present values. This is achieved by attaching declining weights to future events – the further in the future the smaller the weight – and then summing these weighted costs or benefits to produce a present value. Depending on the profile of costs and benefits this can have a marked effect on the attractiveness of different policies or investments.

Consider an intervention that reduces perinatal mortality. A large part of the benefit from such an intervention arises as a stream of future QALYs, many of which are decades in the future. A 60-year life is reduced to 25 years when discounted at a rate of 3.5% (the mechanism will be explained below). To some this may appear to represent an unreasonable biasing of decisions against this group of beneficiaries and in favour of groups where the return is more immediate. But arguably the principle of discounting is simply another recognition of opportunity cost.

Suppose you have £100,000 available to spend on health care and that there are currently opportunities to buy a QALY for £10,000. Assume that such an opportunity is expected to also be available in ten years. If you do not discount future effects you would prefer Project B to Project A (in Table 12.1) – that is, you would prefer an intervention which costs £100,000 now and produces 11 QALYs in ten years to one also costing £100,000 now but producing 10 QALYs this year. Assume that there are opportunities in this economy to invest in productive resources giving a 3.5% real rate of return. Project C involves investing £100,000 now and using the money available as a result in year ten ($£141,000 = £100,000 \, (1.035)^{10}$) to purchase QALYs. Given the possibility of undertaking Project C, the opportunity cost of the 10 QALYs this year which you are giving up in order to obtain 11 QALYs in year ten is

Table 12.1 Three stylized projects

		Benefits	
Project	Action	This year	Year ten
A	Spend £100,000 now on health care	10 QALYs	
B	Spend £100,000 now on health care		11 QALYs
C	Invest £100,000 now and spend £140,000 on health care in year ten		14 QALYs

in fact 14 QALYs in year ten. Thus by not discounting QALYs which accrue in the future you are ignoring opportunity cost and, as a result, would fail to maximize the health benefits.

The lesson of this example is not that you should always be postponing spending on health and investing in the economy instead. Rather, it is that the timing of *when* benefits accrue matters and more specifically, future benefits should be weighted to take account of how far in the future they accrue. Had the benefits from Project B been weighted to allow for their future occurrence it is unlikely that Project B would have been preferred to Project A.

Choosing the discount rate

In practice the choice of discount rate is largely out of your hands and will be determined by the decision-making context, particularly the country in question. However, it is important to have some idea of what lies behind the choice of a discount rate.

Two broad approaches have been put forward for using a positive discount rate: social opportunity cost and social time preference. The social opportunity cost approach emphasizes the opportunity cost in terms of foregone private consumption of investment in the public sector. At its simplest the idea is that investment in the public sector should yield a comparable return to investments in the private sector at the margin. In this case it is the ability of the economy to increase future consumption by postponing current consumption which is determining the discount rate.

The alternative approach is highlighted by current UK government guidance on economic evaluation which stresses the notion of social time preference – that is, the value society attaches to present, as opposed to future, consumption (HM Treasury 2003):

$$r = p + \mu.g$$

where r is the social time preference rate, p is the rate at which future consumption is discounted given no change in per capita consumption, μ the elasticity of marginal utility of consumption with respect to utility and g the annual growth in per capita consumption.

It is suggested that p has two components: a catastrophic risk component and pure time preference. The former describes a situation where some major change occurs which radically alters the expected future returns. The latter captures the preference for consumption now rather than later (independent of any catastrophic risk or anticipation of increasing consumption).

Currently in the UK, ρ is thought to be about 1.5%, μ equal to 1% and g equal to 2%. Putting them all together produces a social time preference rate of 3.5%.

There is a substantial body of evidence suggesting that individuals generally have a positive rate of discount with respect to future health events (Cairns 2001). The estimates vary widely depending to a large extent on the method used to elicit preferences, the time horizon and the nature of the health event.

There has been a certain amount of discussion about whether additional years of life should be discounted at the same rate as future costs or at some lower rate (or possibly be left undiscounted). The present value of life years gained in any particular year can be viewed as the product of three elements: the number of life years gained; the marginal valuation in that year of additional life years; and the weight attached to benefits in that year relative to currently accruing benefits. If life years gained in the future are not discounted but are simply summed, this is equivalent to assuming that the fall in the weight as the life years gained recede into the future is exactly balanced by a rise in the marginal valuation of the additional life years. If the physical quantity of life years gained in any future year is multiplied by the weight implied by the discount rate for costs, this is equivalent to assuming that the marginal valuation of life years remains constant over time. Neither practice will invariably yield the correct answer. Both will involve an element of approximation. All guidelines currently recommend the latter approach – that is, discounting health benefits at the same rate as costs.

Standard discounting model

Interventions with different time profiles of costs and benefits are usually made comparable by discounting future costs and benefits to present values. As noted above, this involves attaching declining weights to future events. In the standard discounting model (variously described as constant rate discounting or exponential discounting) these declining weights or discount factors are equal to $(1+r)^{-t}$ where r is the discount rate and t is the year in which the event occurs. As t increases the discount factor becomes smaller. Letting the discount rate be 0.05, a stream of £1000 either paid or received annually for six years has a present value of £5330 (as shown in Table 12.2).

Table 12.2 Simple illustration of the calculation of present value

	Now	Year 1	Year 2	Year 3	Year 4	Year 5	Total
Amount	£1000	£1000	£1000	£1000	£1000	£1000	£6000
Discount factor	$(1.05)^0$ 1.000	$(1.05)^{-1}$ 0.952	$(1.05)^{-2}$ 0.907	$(1.05)^{-3}$ 0.864	$(1.05)^{-4}$ 0.823	$(1.05)^{-5}$ 0.784	
Present value	£1000	£952	£907	£864	£823	£784	£5330

Essentially what is required of a discounting model is that it should apply a decreasing weight to future costs and effects. There are a very large number of models which can achieve this and so you might ask why is the above model favoured. First, it is simple – it only has a single parameter. Second, it is familiar – it applies in reverse the process of compounding familiar to all with savings. The third reason is more technical. The standard model assumes the axiom of stationarity. This gives the model an attractive normative property, namely that the passage of time *per se* or the point in time at which you make a decision has no effect on which option would be chosen if nothing else has changed. The 'nothing else' includes your estimate of the likely costs and benefits, their timing relative to one another, your budget, other investment opportunities that are available and so on.

Activity 12.1

What is the present value of a stream of ten annual payments of £1000 (1) using a 3% discount rate, and (2) using a 6% discount rate?

Feedback

In practice you would probably use a spreadsheet to calculate present values in an evaluation. But it is important to understand the mechanics of the calculation. The first step would be to identify the discount factors for each year for both discount rates using the formula $(1+r)^{-t}$ and then multiply the payments by these discount factors and add the resulting values together. Thus the discount factors to be applied in the case of a 3% discount rate are 0.9709 in year one, 0.9426 in year two and so on, since 0.9709 equals $(1.03)^{-1}$. The resulting present values are: (1) £8530; and (2) £7360.

Equivalent annual cost

The present value of an annuity (a fixed sum paid or received each year) is given by:

$$PV(a) = a/1+r + a/(1+r)^2 + a/(1+r)^3 + \ldots + a/(1+r)^n$$

There is an arithmetic short-cut (the sum of a geometric series) which lets us re-express this as:

$$PV(a) = a \, (1-1/(1+r)^n/r)$$

The equivalent annual cost (EAC) of any present value is then:

$$a = PV \, / \, (1-1/(1+r)^n/r)$$

For example, suppose a piece of equipment cost £1000 and would last ten years with no scrap value, and assume a discount rate $r = 0.05$.

$$EAC = £1,000/7.7217 \approx £130$$

Note that this is more than the cost divided by the useful life (£100). This is because the equipment will be used for ten years but must be paid for now. The EAC can help the comparison of costs where items such as buildings or equipment have different useful lives.

 Activity 12.2

Suppose that you are refurbishing a building at a cost of £50,000 this year and £25,000 next year and that the building will then have a useful life of 30 years. Calculate the EAC assuming a discount rate r = 0.05.

 Feedback

First express the cost of the refurbishment as a present value

PV = £50,000 + £25,000/1.05 = £73,810

Then estimate the value of $(1-1/(1.05)^{30}/0.05) = 15.373$

EAC = £73,810/15.373 = £4,801

Does discounting make a difference?

When comparing mutually exclusive interventions with similar profiles in terms of the timing of costs and effects, the choice of discount rate (and whether you discount at all) is unlikely to make any difference to which project is selected. However, when these time profiles differ the use of a discount rate and its particular value can play a significant role in determining which project is preferred. This is perhaps clearest when considering immediate treatment versus prevention. Suppose you are considering the development of a cardiovascular strategy. Almost certainly you would want to have a combination of policies, including treatment and prevention. However, since the budget is inevitably limited it is likely that you will want to know what additional spending on surgery (such as coronary artery bypass grafts) brings as compared to additional spending on cholesterol-lowering drugs. The benefits of surgery will start immediately but will also stretch into the future. The benefits of cholesterol-lowering drugs will take longer to accrue but will also continue for longer. The costs of surgery are largely early on whereas the costs of cholesterol-lowering drugs are spread more evenly over time. The higher the discount rate, other things being equal, prevention becomes less attractive relative to surgery.

Another example would be the choice between a vaccination programme to prevent future disease and a treatment programme for existing cases. Other things being equal, the higher the discount rate the less attractive is a preventive policy, since the benefits tend to be further in the future relative to the costs than is the case with a treatment programme.

Another situation where discounting will potentially be important is when decision-making is influenced by cost-effectiveness thresholds. Since many interventions tend to be characterized by substantial initial costs but benefits in the future, the use of discounting tends to make the project appear less attractive,

Table 12.3 Antenatal screening for hepatitis B

	Universal screening	Selective screening
Screening costs	£366,000	£91,000
Vaccination and immunoglobulin costs	£223,000	£168,000
Saving in treatment costs	£114,000	£86,000
Net cost	£475,000	£173,000
Life years gained	529.7 years	397.3 years
Discounted life years gained	42.7 years	32.0 years
Cost per life year gained	£900	£450
Cost per discounted life year gained	£11,000	£5400

Source: Adapted from Tormans et al. (1993)

particularly if there is a substantial delay before most of the benefits accrue. This is illustrated in Table 12.3. The costs of screening, and the vaccination and immuno-globulin costs, are incurred when the programme is implemented. There will be some cost saving with respect to future treatment (which you can assume has been suitably discounted). Because the life years gained largely accrue once the children of the mothers in the programme reach middle age, discounting has a dramatic impact reducing the 529.7 life years gained by universal screening to a present value of 42.7 years. This clearly has a marked effect on the estimated cost-effectiveness of the programme.

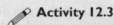 **Activity 12.3**

Suppose there is a choice between the three projects shown in Table 12.4.

Table 12.4 Comparison of three projects

	Project A		Project B		Project C	
	Cost	QALYs	Cost	QALYs	Cost	QALYs
Yr 0	£20,000		£20,000		£10,000	
Yr 1	£20,000	1 QALY	£20,000		£10,000	0.5 QALY
Yr 2	£20,000	1 QALY	£20,000		£10,000	0.5 QALY
Yr 3		1 QALY			£10,000	0.5 QALY
Yr 4		1 QALY			£10,000	0.5 QALY
Yr 5					£10,000	0.5 QALY
Yr 6						0.5 QALY
Yr 7						0.5 QALY
Yr 8						0.5 QALY
Yr 9				1 QALY		
Yr 10				1 QALY		
Yr 11				1 QALY		
Yr 12				1 QALY		

Before doing any discounting, order the projects in terms of cost per QALY. Then re-express as present values using a discount rate of 5% and calculate the cost per QALY. Assume the figures above are all incremental costs and incremental QALYs compared to current practice.

Feedback

In the absence of any discounting all projects have a cost per QALY of £15,000. With a 5% discount rate the costs per QALY are (A) £16,128, (B) £23,828 and (C) £16,492.

Intergenerational equity

The use of any positive discount rate given a sufficiently long time period over which to operate will generate very small present values no matter how large is the distant cost or effect. As a result it is sometimes suggested that discounting is unfair to future generations. The present generation may under-invest in projects with very large returns to future generations because these returns are not so very large when expressed as present values. Similarly, the present generation may in its decision-making attach a rather small weight to very large future costs bequeathed to future generations. These considerations are sometimes used to suggest that discounting is inappropriate.

One potential solution is to distinguish between intragenerational and intergenerational discounting. For the reasons already advanced in this chapter, discounting within a generation is argued to be appropriate but having discounted each generation's costs and benefits to its own present value, these present values should be combined by use of equity weights. These weights reflect the current generation's altruism towards future generations. Consider the evaluation of a programme to eradicate a disease. Discounting the future benefits back to the present day would result in a very small weight being attached to the benefits several hundred years in the future from eradication of the disease. If instead the present value of disease eradication to each future generation were added together using equity weights, it is likely that the programme would appear much more attractive to the present generation.

Another potential solution is to have discount factors which fall as the time horizon lengthens but do not fall as rapidly as implied by the standard constant rate discounting model. Recent theoretical developments have supported such an approach. Recent guidance in the UK now recommends time varying discount rates, namely 3.5% (years 0 to 30), 3.0% (years 31 to 75), 2.5% (years 76 to 125), 2.0% (years 126 to 200), 1.5% (years 201 to 300) and 1% thereafter (HM Treasury 2003). Most health care interventions that have been assessed to date have a time horizon of less than 50 years and thus would not be influenced by this change in practice.

Discounting practice

All guidelines regarding the conduct of economic evaluation require discounting (whenever the costs and effects are not restricted to the near future). While the actual rate of discount recommended varies to some extent between countries, the use of the standard discounting model is universal, and the same rate of discount is applied to both the costs and the benefits, even when the latter are expressed in non-monetary form such as life years or QALYs.

While countries differ with respect to the rate of discount that they recommend for use in the analysis of the base case, most recommend between 3 and 5%. There are exceptions. For example, New Zealand uses 10%, the influential Washington Panel recommended 3% (Gold *et al.* 1996) and a similar rate is built into DALY estimations. In addition, the guidelines in most countries recommend examining the impact of discounting in a sensitivity analysis (see Chapter 14). Several guidelines also recommend reporting undiscounted costs and effects.

For a number of years practice in England and Wales provided a unique exception to this uniformity. Costs were discounted at 6% and QALYs at 1.5%. This practical exception arose because the view was taken that the arguments put forward for discounting costs and effects at the same rate were not compelling and that a case could be made for a lower rate in the case of health benefits. However, the recommended rate is now 3.5% for both costs and health benefits (HM Treasury 2003).

Activity 12.4

Assess the case for and against discounting future costs and effects in the economic evaluation of health care interventions.

Feedback

The case for discounting can be made either with respect to the opportunity cost of foregone private consumption, or with respect to the value that society attaches to present as opposed to future consumption. A case against discounting might possibly be made in terms of intergenerational equity, and the introduction of systematic bias if the wrong rate is chosen. Some authors have argued that health is different and should be treated differently in terms of discounting (Parsonage and Neuburger 1992).

Summary

You have learnt about the need to discount costs and how this is commonly done. You saw the impact that discounting can have on decisions and the debate about whether or not to also discount benefits. That completes the section of the book on measuring and valuing consequences. It is time to consider the presentation and interpretation of economic evidence.

References

Cairns JA (2001) Discounting in economic evaluation, in M Drummond and A McGuire (eds) *Economic evaluation in health care: merging theory with practice*. Oxford: Oxford University Press.

Gold MR, Siegel JE, Russell LB and Weinstein MC (eds) (1996) *Cost-effectiveness in health and medicine*. Oxford: Oxford University Press.

HM Treasury (2003) *The Green Book: appraisal and evaluation in central government*. London: The Stationery Office.

Parsonage M and Neuburger H (1992) Discounting and health benefits. *Health Economics* 1:71–6.

Tormans G, Van Damme P, Carrin G, Clara R and Eylenbusch W (1993) Cost-effectiveness analysis of perinatal screening and vaccination against hepatitis B virus – the case of Belgium. *Social Science and Medicine* 37:173–81.

Further reading

A very useful website which provides details on the guidelines for more than 20 countries has been provided by the International Society for Pharmacoeconomics and Outcomes Research (www.ispor.org/PEguidelines/index.asp).

SECTION 4

Presenting and interpreting the evidence

13 Interpreting incremental cost-effectiveness ratios

Overview

This is the first of four chapters on presenting and interpreting evidence. Incremental cost-effectiveness ratios (ICERs) are the summary measures used to report the cost-effectiveness of different interventions. This chapter focuses on how ICERs can be used to inform decision-making with respect to mutually exclusive and independent health care programmes.

Learning objectives

After working through this chapter, you will be able to:

- **interpret results presented in a cost-effectiveness plane**
- **use ICERs to compare the cost-effectiveness of different interventions**
- **understand the concepts of dominance and extended dominance**
- **allocate a fixed budget so as to maximize the number of QALYs produced**

Key terms

Cost-effectiveness acceptability curve A method of graphically displaying the results from a probabilistic sensitivity analysis.

Cost-effectiveness plane A figure with which incremental costs and incremental effects can be plotted relative to a comparator.

Cost-effectiveness threshold The level of cost per unit of outcome below which an intervention might be described as cost-effective.

Dominance When one intervention is both less costly and more effective than the comparators

Extended dominance When one intervention is both less costly and more effective than a linear combination of two other interventions with which it is mutually exclusive.

Mutually exclusive interventions When implementation of a particular intervention excludes the possibility of implementing other interventions – for example, if one drug is used as first-line treatment for a particular condition this implies that any other drug cannot be used as first-line treatment.

Threshold analysis The value of a parameter is varied to find the level at which the results change (e.g. the level at which the cost per DALY reaches $50).

Cost-effectiveness plane

A cost-effectiveness plane is a useful construction for comparing two or more interventions (see Figure 13.1). The horizontal axis by convention measures differences in effectiveness and the vertical axis measures differences in costs. Suppose you are comparing an old and a new treatment for a particular condition. Ignoring the possibility that they do not differ with respect to costs or effects there are four possibilities. The four quadrants can be identified as in a map. In the north-east quadrant the new treatment is more effective but also costs more. In the south-east quadrant the new treatment dominates the old treatment. In the south-west quadrant the new treatment is less effective but it is also less costly. Finally, in the north-west quadrant the old treatment dominates the new treatment. Interpretation is self-evident in the SE and NW quadrants assuming that all relevant differences in costs and in effects have been captured.

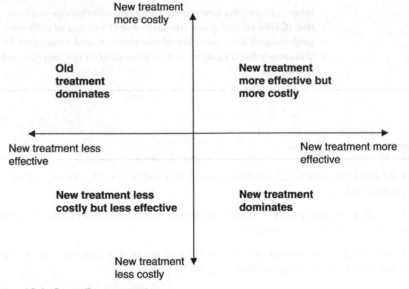

Figure 13.1 Cost-effectiveness plane

The NE quadrant is where attention is more often focused. Here the issue is how the additional effect compares to the additional cost. However, note that essentially the same issue arises in the SW quadrant – how does the cost saving compare to the loss of effectiveness? There is often a reluctance to consider a new treatment unless it has the prospect of being more effective than existing treatments (whatever it costs). If you label the treatments A and B rather than old and new, and if you measure the effectiveness of A minus the effectiveness of B on the horizontal axis and the cost of A minus the cost of B on the vertical axis, any points that were in the SW quadrant are now in the NE quadrant. The question again seems to be, how does the additional cost compare with the additional benefit (and few would argue that you should ignore the cost difference)?

Incremental cost-effectiveness ratios

The results from CEAs and CUAs are presented as incremental cost-effectiveness ratios (ICERs) in the form of:

$$\frac{\text{Total cost of new intervention} - \text{total cost of old intervention}}{\text{Outcome of new intervention} - \text{outcome of old intervention}}$$

Replacing 'outcome' with QALYs would give an ICER for a CUA. This way of expressing the results highlights the importance of the choice of comparators referred to Chapter 4. A new intervention can often be made to appear cost-effective through the choice of an inappropriate comparator.

The slope of a ray from the origin to any point is equal to the $\Delta C/\Delta QALY$ (see Figure 13.2). Thus each point in the cost-effectiveness plane represents an ICER. In Figure 13.2 all combinations of incremental QALYs and incremental costs that lie on the same ray from the origin have the same ICER. The steeper the slope the higher the ratio and the less cost-effective the intervention relative to the comparator.

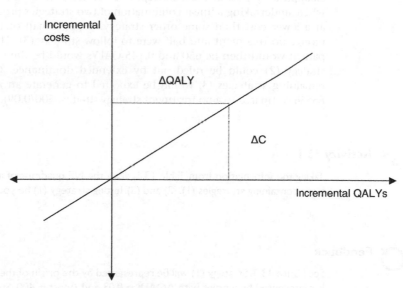

Figure 13.2 Incremental cost-effectiveness ratio

Dominance and extended dominance

You have already come across dominance graphically (points lying in the SE and NW quadrants) in the cost-effectiveness plane. Consider a comparison of different treatment strategies shown in Table 13.1. The comparator is no treatment. There are assumed to be two drugs, A and B. Drug A could be tried and continued until there is no evidence of an effect or evidence of an adverse reaction and similarly for Drug B. Alternatively, one drug could be tried first and in the event that there was no beneficial effect (or if there was an adverse reaction) the other drug could be tried.

Table 13.1 Treatment strategies ordered by increasing cost

Strategy	Cost	QALY	
1) No additional treatment	400	0.10	
2) Drug B – no treatment	800	0.13	Dominated by a combination of (1) and (3)
3) Drug B – Drug A – no treatment	900	0.19	5556 per QALY
4) Drug A – no treatment	1000	0.17	Dominated by (3)
5) Drug A – Drug B – no treatment	1100	0.18	Dominated by (3)

The strategies are ordered in terms of increasing cost in Table 13.1. By doing this it is straightforward to identify dominated strategies – cases where the cost rises but effectiveness declines. Note strategies (4) and (5) are dominated by strategy (3). This example also illustrates the concept of extended dominance. This is the situation where undertaking a linear combination of two strategies produces a greater effect at a lower cost than some other strategy. Suppose half of the patients were to receive no treatment and half were to follow strategy (3). The expected cost per patient would then be 650 and 0.145 QALYs would be the expected effect. Thus strategy (2) could be ruled out by extended dominance. Comparing the two remaining strategies (3) would be expected to generate an additional QALY for £5556 compared to a no treatment strategy (that is, 500/0.09).

Activity 13.1

Taking the information from Table 13.1, draw the NE quadrant of a cost-effectiveness plane containing strategies (1), (2) and (3), letting strategy (1) be your comparator.

Feedback

See Figure 13.3. Strategy (1) will be represented by the origin of the graph. Strategy (2) is represented by a point with ΔQALY = 0.03 and Δcost = 400. Strategy (3) is represented by a point with ΔQALY = 0.09 and Δcost = 500. A ray from the origin to point (3), which represents cost-effectiveness, could be achieved by combinations of strategies (1) and (3), has several points SE of point (2). This illustrates extended dominance graphically.

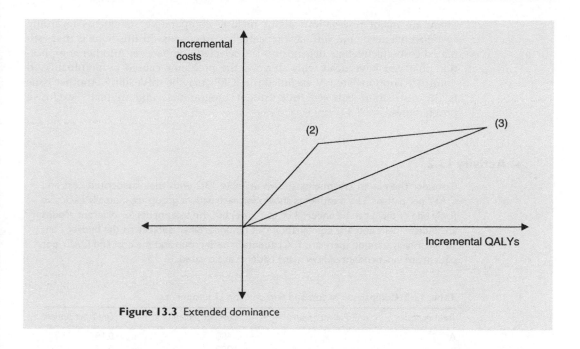

Figure 13.3 Extended dominance

Cost-effectiveness thresholds

How can you determine whether or not a particular intervention is cost-effective in the sense of representing a good use of scarce health care resources given the other opportunities available? If the effects could be re-expressed in monetary terms it would be possible to identify whether or not the more cost-effective of the two interventions did represent a good use of resources by comparing costs and effects directly. As identified in Chapter 10, there are a number of challenges raised by monetary valuation of health outcomes and so, generally, the information available to decision-makers will at best be in terms of cost per QALY. There is a strong temptation to rank interventions in terms of ascending cost per QALY (so-called QALY league tables) starting with the lowest cost per QALY activity. There are a number of problems with such an approach not least that it doesn't reflect the incremental nature of real-world decision-making and that decisions are being made more or less continuously rather than at the start of a five-year plan. The notion of cost-effectiveness thresholds has been introduced to help determine whether particular ICERs indicate whether an intervention represents a good use of resources. The appeal is obvious: it appears to permit decisions to be taken as and when they arise. Also, assuming that the threshold is explicit, it adds to the transparency of decision-making.

But how do you decide at what level to set the threshold? The threshold should reflect the size of the budget and the other opportunities available for using these scarce resources. Some authors argue strongly that it is necessary to identify not just the cost-effectiveness of any new option under consideration but also the cost-effectiveness of the activity that will be displaced.

There are major reservations about making comparative statements regarding cost-effectiveness. One you have repeatedly come across in this book is that estimated cost-effectiveness depends on the selected comparator. Another complication that you have dealt with above is the problems caused by dominance. If dominated options are not excluded the ICERs may be misleading. Another issue is the distinction between independent programmes and mutually exclusive programmes.

Activity 13.2

Consider the eleven treatments shown in Table 13.2 with their associated cost and QALY per patient. The treatments shown for each patient group are mutually exclusive (only one of them can be undertaken at a time) but the treatments for different groups are independent and any combination can be undertaken subject to the budget constraint. Finally, assume there are 100 patients in each group and the cost and QALY per patient are independent of how many patients are treated.

Table 13.2 Comparison of cost and outcome for 11 treatments

Treatment	Patient group	Cost per patient	QALY per patient
A	1	400	0.10
B	1	1000	0.17
C	1	800	0.13
D	1	1100	0.18
E	1	900	0.19
F	2	200	0.05
G	2	400	0.08
H	2	600	0.12
I	3	100	0.03
J	3	450	0.06
K	3	300	0.05

1   Identify dominated treatments.
2   What are the maximum number of QALYs which can be achieved with a budget of
    (a) £70,000, (b) £120,000 and (c) £180,000?
3   How large would your budget have to be for treatment K to appear cost-effective?

Feedback

1 Treatments B and D produce fewer QALYs at a higher cost than treatment E. Treatment C is dominated by a combination of treatments A and E. Treatment G is dominated by a combination of treatments F and H.

2 Start by purchasing the treatment with the lowest ICER and add treatments for other patient groups as the budget permits or substitute more effective treatments for a particular patient group again as the budget permits. QALYs will be maximized as follows: (a) purchase A, F and I, (b) purchase E, F and I, (c) purchase E, H and I.

3 Treatment K will only become attractive once the budget exceeds £168,000. At that point it becomes worthwhile replacing treatment I by treatment K.

The example above involved a known and fixed budget, and considered how to maximize the health gain from a given level of spending. The other situation in which cost-effectiveness thresholds are used is as an aid to decision-making by national bodies, such as NICE in England and Wales, when deciding on whether or not to recommend the adoption of particular health technologies. In such circumstances the precise budget is not specified and any cost-effectiveness threshold is necessarily less explicit because of greater uncertainty about the opportunity cost of any programmes that would be displaced as a result of any adoption decision.

Thus NICE does not use a fixed ICER threshold in the sense that technologies with an ICER below this value will definitely be accepted and those with a higher ICER will be rejected. It does, however, make reference in its guidance to a cost-effectiveness threshold of £20,000/QALY. Above this 'judgements about the acceptability of the technology as an effective use of NHS resources are more likely to make more explicit reference to factors including: the degree of uncertainty surrounding the calculation of ICERs; the innovative nature of the technology; the particular features of the condition and population receiving the technology; and where appropriate, the wider societal costs and benefits'. And for ICERs above £30,000/QALY 'the case for supporting the technology on these factors has to be increasingly strong' (NICE 2004).

Confidence intervals

In practice there are large uncertainties regarding much of the information required in order to estimate ICERs. As a result it is widely accepted that a simple point estimate of an ICER (mean incremental cost divided by mean incremental effectiveness) is unlikely to be adequate information with which to inform decision-making. One response to these uncertainties is to undertake sensitivity analyses and this is dealt with in Chapters 14 and 15. Another response has been to place confidence intervals around the ICER estimates.

Many economic evaluations lack individual data on resource use and instead use estimates based on average or representative patients. The cost estimate has no variance and so a confidence interval for the costs (or for the ICER) cannot be calculated. However, as increasingly data are generated in trials with effects and costs for individual patients the scope for estimating confidence intervals for ICERs has been increased. One major complication is that, unlike a confidence interval for an effect size or for a difference in costs, it involves estimating a confidence interval for a ratio (the denominator of which can on occasion be zero). One issue of considerable concern has been the nature of the correlation between costs and effects. This correlation has a major impact on the size of the confidence interval.

Non-parametric bootstrapping has been advocated as a potential solution to the unknown sampling distribution of the ICER. This approach builds an estimate of the sampling distribution by re-sampling (with replacement) the original distribution. Once this empirical estimate has been constructed it is straight-forward to estimate confidence limits, for example, using the percentile method. Interest in confidence intervals for ICERs has to some extent waned with the rise of probabilistic sensitivity analysis (see Chapter 15).

Summary

You have learnt about how to compare the cost-effectiveness of rival interventions using a simple cost-effectiveness plane. This helps demonstrate dominance and extended dominance. You went on to look at cost-effectiveness thresholds and the uncertainties around estimates of ICERs.

References

NICE (2004) *Guide to methods of technology appraisal*. London: NICE, www.nice.org.uk/pdf/TAP_Methods.pdf.

Further reading

Briggs AH (2001) Handling uncertainty in economic evaluation and presenting the results, in M Drummond and A McGuire (eds) *Economic evaluation in health care: merging theory with practice*. Oxford: Oxford University Press.

Manning WG, Fryback DG and Weinstein MC (1996) Reflecting uncertainty in cost-effectiveness analysis, in MR Gold *et al.* (eds) *Cost-effectiveness in health and medicine*. Oxford: Oxford University Press.

14 | Basic sensitivity analysis

Overview

When data are collected and/or assumptions are made within an economic evaluation, uncertainty arises as to the accuracy of these parameters and therefore the emphasis that can be placed on the resulting cost-effectiveness estimate. The impact of this uncertainty can (and should) be assessed by undertaking a sensitivity analysis. You will learn about the types of uncertainty that can arise in an economic evaluation and be provided with suggestions on how to plan a sensitivity analysis. A number of specific techniques are worked through with examples, followed by a discussion of when it is best to use them and the advantages and disadvantages of each approach.

Learning objectives

After working through this chapter, you will be able to:

- **identify the sources of uncertainty**
- **understand what sensitivity analysis is**
- **understand the advantages and disadvantages of different approaches**
- **undertake a one-way and multi-way sensitivity analysis**

Key terms

Multi-way (multivariate) sensitivity analysis An exploration of the impact on the results of changing the value of two or more parameters at the same time.

One-way (univariate) sensitivity analysis An exploration of the impact on the results of changing the value of one parameter while keeping the values of all other parameters unchanged.

Parameter uncertainty The acknowledgement that a precise value of a parameter is not always known. This is also referred to as 'second order' uncertainty. It is represented in an analysis by specifying variables as distributions.

Reference case A set of assumptions and methods which should wherever possible be followed by all economic evaluations so that different studies can be more readily compared.

Scenario analysis A form of multi-way sensitivity analysis, such as setting all parameters at their most favourable or unfavourable values in order to find how low or high the incremental cost-effectiveness ratio becomes.

Uncertainty, ultimately with regard to the precision of the ICER, is inherent in any economic evaluation. Briggs and Gray (1999) identify three broad areas of uncertainty.

Methodological uncertainty

This relates to the general methods used within an economic evaluation and includes issues such as the methods used to identify, measure and value costs and health consequences. For instance, it is known that different methods of elicitation can produce different utility estimates (as you learnt in Chapter 9). Another common example of this type of uncertainty concerns the extrapolation of the results of randomized trials; what statistical function should be fitted to observed data in order to predict longer-term consequences?

A related issue surrounds the use of decision modelling in economic evaluation. By definition, this approach requires the analyst to construct and link up a series of mathematical or statistical equations to estimate cost-effectiveness, but it is easy to make mistakes when doing this as the programming can be complex. Sensitivity analysis can be used to test the internal logic of the programming. For example, if a hazard ratio (the rate of an event with treatment to the rate of an event without treatment) is used to estimate the relative treatment effects of a technology, then all else being equal, the treatments should be equally effective when this value is set to 1. If not, then it is likely something is awry with the programming.

The 'reference case' approach is one method of addressing this type of uncertainty, which you will learn more about in Chapter 16. It involves specifying a core set of methodological assumptions that should be common across all economic evaluations. However, the remaining uncertainty associated with the effects of applying different parameter estimates can only be handled using different tools, and the reference case requires that additional sensitivity analysis be undertaken. It is important to note also that the reference case has yet to be validated for low- and middle-income countries.

Uncertainty in data requirements

Variability within different populations with respect to data on costs and health consequences is a key source of uncertainty. For example, unit costs can vary by supplier. The question becomes which is the most appropriate value to use in the analysis – often there is no 'correct' answer (unless all values are identical). Another example is the use of capital equipment. A cost per patient will be a function of the rate at which the value of the capital depreciates. However, what is the appropriate depreciation rate when its mean life span is unknown?

Generalizability

Among other issues, an economic evaluation should be clear in terms of the patient group to which it relates, the resources it includes and the context to which it applies. Generalizability refers to the extent to which the results can be applied to different settings, such as different patient groups and contexts. For example, the costs per patient of being treated with a piece of capital equipment will, all else being equal, decrease as more patients are treated with it. Therefore, a useful sensitivity analysis could assess the impact of varying patient numbers in a given time period and make useful comments regarding the most cost-effective location for the equipment. Technology that does not appear to be cost-effective in areas with few patients may well be when located in a busier clinic.

How to perform a basic sensivitiy analysis

The following three extracts from Walker and Fox-Rushby (2001) describe how to perform a basic sensitivity analysis.

 Getting started: planning the sensitivity analysis

There are several steps that need to be performed prior to undertaking any type of sensitivity analysis. For each type of uncertainty (for costs and consequences) analysts need to:

1 Identify all the parameters or approaches to modelling that could be subjected to sensitivity analysis (in principle the model and all parameters are potential candidates);
2 Choose the input parameters or approaches to modelling that you feel are most important to subject to a sensitivity analysis from the list of possibilities, and provide a justification for the choices made. For example, you may consider those variables (for the quantity or price/value of costs and effects) that:

   • are the most uncertain;
   • have the greatest sampling variability;
   • are based on the weakest quality evidence, such as assumptions;
   • are most in the control of policy-makers;
   • influence the largest percentage of total cost/effects;
   • are more likely to differ from published data;
   • are subject to greatest disagreements regarding methods;
   • are key to explaining how costs and/or effects vary across settings.

   Analysts should also justify why some parameters, if any, or different types of models, have not been subjected to sensitivity analysis (for example, because the parameter is known with certainty or will only have a minimal impact on results).
3 Choose the range of alternative values or models that you will substitute into the base-case analysis, providing a justification for all choices made for both the size and direction of this change. The range of values adopted may be drawn from the literature, expert opinion accessed through consensus building techniques, sampling variation in the original data, or the researcher's own views. For parameter uncertainty, the following might be considered:

   • for deterministic data – high and low values of each key variable;
   • for stochastic data – the range, plus or minus one standard deviation of sampling

error from clinical data, or the most often used 95% confidence intervals for key parameters to determine a plausible range for variation.

For modelling uncertainty, the following might be considered:

* using alternative functional forms for key variables;
* including/excluding particular types of costs/effects;
* asking another person/group to undertake the analysis starting with the same initial information;
* using a different model structure.

4 Choose which techniques to use to analyse uncertainty (see the next section on techniques of sensitivity analysis) and apply the sensitivity analysis to the evaluation. We suggest beginning with one-way analyses as a route to understanding the impact of individual variables/models prior to moving to multivariate analyses.

5 The final step in a sensitivity analysis is to interpret the findings. The analyst must determine how much change from the base-case result is acceptable or constitutes a robust finding and/or the combination of parameter values required to achieve pre-determined incremental cost-effectiveness ratios. Typically, the key question to ask yourself is whether the results from the sensitivity analysis are sufficient to change the decision at hand.

 Activity 14.1

Suppose you have been asked to evaluate the cost-effectiveness of intermittent preventive treatment with anti-malaria drugs to reduce anaemia and malaria morbidity in children. Identify five examples of parameter uncertainty which it might be advisable to consider in any sensitivity analysis.

 Feedback

There are many possible answers including: effectiveness of preventive treatment; length and intensity of seasonal malaria transmission; cost of preventive treatment; cost of treating anaemia and malaria morbidity; frequency of side-effects; health benefits of reductions in anaemia and malaria.

 Techniques of sensitivity analyses

This section describes the different types of sensitivity analysis that are available. The predominant focus is on approaches to estimating the impact of parameter uncertainty in one-way and multi-way sensitivity analysis using worked examples. All examples focus on treating pregnant women with antiretroviral therapy to reduce mother-to-child transmission of HIV and are purely illustrative.

One-way (univariate) sensitivity analysis

The traditional approach to sensitivity analysis is to examine the impact on an ICER of changing one variable at a time. This is known as one-way or univariate sensitivity analysis (Table 14.1). The process is simple: after calculating the base-case scenario, the incremental

Table 14.1 Example of one-way sensitivity analysis

	HIV seroprevalence among pregnant women	ICER	% divergence from base case
Low value	15%	$53	+36%
Base-case estimate	20%	$39	–
High value	25%	$32	−18%

Source: Walker and Fox-Rushby (2001)

cost-effectiveness ratio is re-calculated holding all parameters constant apart from the parameter selected to vary over a specified (and justified) range. This process is repeated for as many parameters as desired, and ideally all of the model parameters. However, it is important to remember to reset the analysis back to the base-case after each sensitivity analysis to ensure that only one variable at a time is changed (relative to the base-case). When a small change in the input parameter causes a large change to the ICER, the ICER is said to be 'sensitive' to that variable. However, when a large change in the input variable causes only a small change to the ICER, it is said to be 'robust' to change.

A second type of one-way analysis is a 'threshold analysis'. This concept is drawn from decision analysis, where the analyst varies the size of an input parameter over a range and determines the level above or below which the conclusions change, and hence the 'threshold' point at which neither of the alternatives are favoured over the other. Threshold analysis could be used to (say) assess the incremental survival required to produce an ICER of a given (and fixed) amount. Often this given amount will reflect an ICER above which the technology would not be considered cost-effective. The important point to note in this example is that it is no longer the ICER that is being generated, indeed the ICER is being held constant, it is the size of the incremental survival sufficient to produce an ICER of a given amount that is being estimated.

Relative to the other techniques described, one-way sensitivity analysis is easy to do and provides flexibility in parameter choice. It is a logical, straightforward place to start to understand the structure of a particular cost-effectiveness analysis and provides the building blocks to perform multi-way sensitivity analyses. Also, by determining the variables to which the ICER is sensitive, it can shed light on whether any additional research could improve the outcome from a policy decision and whether it is worth waiting for these additional data.

Although insightful, one-way sensitivity analyses (by themselves) are inadequate. Examining one source of uncertainty at a time provides an incomplete picture and an underestimation of how uncertain the results actually are (Agro et al. 1997). There are three related problems:

- the incremental cost and effectiveness depend on multiple parameters, not just one;
- the interaction of particular factors may imply that the total effect is quite different from the simple sum of individual contributions (sometimes referred to as non-linearity);
- the cost-effectiveness ratio is a ratio of two uncertain numbers, with the result that the uncertainty in the ratio may be substantially larger than that of either of its elements.

Multi-way (multivariate) sensitivity analysis

In one-way sensitivity analysis, the value of parameters are changed one at a time. In multi-way analysis the value of two or more parameters are changed simultaneously. It recognises that more than one parameter value within an evaluation may be uncertain.

For a two-way analysis, the first step is to construct a two-by-two matrix reflecting the incremental cost-effectiveness for every combination of the two variables of interest. Table 14.2 shows how the estimated cost per DALY averted for different combinations of the price of antiretroviral therapy and seroprevalence. The second step is to identify the pairs of values that equalise a pre-determined willingness-to-pay for a unit of effect, i.e. the values of the two variables at which the ICER equals the threshold value. Suppose $60 is the maximum sum that a government is willing to pay to avert a DALY. The combinations of price and seroprevalence that produce this threshold cost-effectiveness ratio can be identified and presented graphically. In Figure 14.1 the six combinations yielding $60 per DALY averted are plotted and a curve is drawn through them. Combinations of price and seroprevalence above the line would then not be regarded as cost-effective, whereas combinations below the line are regarded as cost-effective.

Table 14.2 Example of two-way sensitivity analysis

	Price of antiretroviral therapy ($)									
Seroprevalence	0.17	0.25	0.50	0.62	0.75	0.84	0.98	1.00	1.07	1.13
10%	**60**	65	72	80	97	110	125	150	172	200
15%	25	33	45	**60**	75	90	110	130	150	170
20%	15	17	20	45	52	**60**	75	90	110	130
25%	12	15	17	20	45	55	**60**	85	90	110
30%	10	12	15	17	20	30	45	50	**60**	85
35%	7	10	12	15	17	22	30	45	55	**60**
40%	5	7	10	12	15	20	25	30	35	45

Source: Walker and Fox-Rushby (2001)

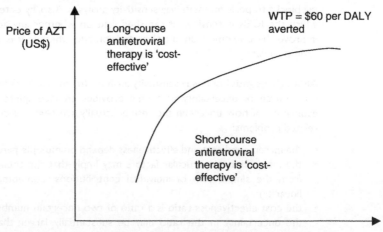

Figure 14.1 Graphical illustration of two-way sensitivity analysis

Source: Walker and Fox-Rushby (2001)

Another type of multi-way sensitivity analysis is 'scenario analysis', of which there are many examples. There are also a variety of approaches that can be used to develop scenarios that encompass the researcher thinking through possible scenarios themselves, through to scenarios developed with consensus group techniques. We note three types of scenarios that might be used:

- analysis of the set of extreme circumstances across parameters, also known as 'worst/best' case analysis. In the worst (best) case scenario the parameter values that yield the highest (lowest) cost-effectiveness ratios are combined;
- use of an agreed 'reference case' of methods by analysts. The most well known reference case is set out by Gold et al. (1996) which sets out the methodological guidance from the report of the Panel on Cost-Effectiveness and Medicine in the United States. It is particularly aimed at increasing the quality and comparability of results across interventions and reducing what has been described as 'methodological uncertainty';
- evaluating all cost-effectiveness ratios alongside a scenario assuming no interventions at all (Hutubessy et al. 2003). This involves the development of natural history models to estimate the impact of disease without any formal sector health care interventions and redefining all interventions considered with respect to this null set. It is argued that this approach will increase the generalisability of results across regions of the world.

Functional form sensitivity analysis is related to both one- and multi-way sensitivity analysis. However, it can be given a separate mention because it is an explicit recognition that one- and multi-way analyses have traditionally not tended to question the way that parameters are assumed to be related to each other in an underlying disease model. Computing incremental cost-effectiveness ratios using different types of models and comparing the impact on the final ratios is the only approach recommended to date (Manning et al. 1996). The two main approaches to this are either for the analyst to re-run models or for different analysts or groups of analysts to run their own models on the same data. Examples of some of the structural issues that could be considered include:

- comparing simple and more complex models (e.g. judging the impact of increasing the ability to distinguish different types of patients);
- comparing the effect of using multiplicative or additive models of diseases, interventions evaluated and co-morbidities when calculating age-sex specific hazard functions.

The advantage of multi-way sensitivity analysis is that it produces more realistic results than one-way sensitivity analysis. Two- and three-way sensitivity analyses can be helpful to identify the best scenario likely to appeal to decision-makers with a note of the reliability of such a situation, but they also suffer from some of the same problems of one-way sensitivity analyses; namely, that they may be difficult to interpret if the variables used are dependent on each other (Agro et al. 1997). However, multi-way becomes increasingly time-consuming to perform as the possible combinations of different parameters increases and is of less use if the results are sensitive to the extreme combinations of parameter values (Agro et al. 1997).

The variety of univariate and multivariate sensitivity analyses provide a range of complementary techniques for dealing with uncertainty. You will strengthen your evaluation of health care programmes by performing a range of sensitivity analyses in order to best capture the extent to which uncertainty is present in your findings, and hence the robustness of your results and recommendations.

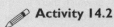

Activity 14.2

Suppose a particular condition is currently treated using treatment A and a new treatment B has been proposed. The expected total cost and total QALYs expected per patient are shown in Table 14.3.

Table 14.3 Expected total cost and total QALYs per patient

Annual drug cost for treatment B	200	250	300	350	400
Total cost for treatment A	400	400	400	400	400
Total cost for treatment B	400	450	500	550	600
Response to treatment A	0.15	0.20	0.25	0.30	0.35
Total QALYs from treatment A	0.030	0.038	0.045	0.051	0.056
Response to treatment B	0.20	0.25	0.30	0.35	0.40
Total QALYs from treatment B	0.035	0.045	0.050	0.055	0.060

1   Assuming a base case of response to treatment A (B) = 0.25 (0.30) and total cost of treatment A (B) = 400 (500), calculate the ICER for the comparison of treatment B with treatment A.
2   How sensitive is this estimate to the assumed annual medication cost for treatment B?
3   Present a two-way sensitivity analysis with respect to the assumed response to treatment A and treatment B.

Feedback

1   Δcost/ΔQALYs = £100/0.005 = £20,000.

2   Calculate the ICER for each annual cost of drug B:

Annual cost	£200	£250	£300	£350	£400
	B dominates A	£10,000	£20,000	£30,000	£40,000

3   The comparison of treatment B with treatment A produces the ICERs for different combinations of responses to treatment shown in Table 14.4.

Table 14.4 ICERs for different combinations of responses to treatment

Response to treatment B	Response to treatment A				
	0.15	0.20	0.25	0.30	0.35
0.20	£20,000	A dominates	A dominates	A dominates	A dominates
0.25	£6667	£14,286	A dominates	A dominates	A dominates
0.30	£5000	£8333	£20,000	A dominates	A dominates
0.35	£4000	£5882	£10,000	£25,000	A dominates
0.40	£3333	£4545	£6667	£11,111	£25,000

How should the results of sensitivity analysis be interpreted?

Having set out why sensitivity analysis is needed, and how it might be planned and executed, it is important to consider how the results of sensitivity analyses might be interpreted.

The first step is to note which variables cause the greatest and least change in the incremental cost-effectiveness ratio. Two main difficulties arise: what constitutes a large/small change; and how likely is such a change. With a sensitivity analysis both these decisions are the analyst's own judgement and the basis of such decisions needs to be open for readers (and policy-makers) to assess and consider changing according to different views about the future. The analyst makes a judgement of how likely this is to be and therefore how robust conclusions about the base-case results are. Ultimately, however, the real test is to understand whether different assumptions alter the decision being addressed.

The implications of the results of the sensitivity analysis can be considered in terms of recommendations for policy and/or research. For example:

- results of a sensitivity analysis may show that reducing uncertainty by collecting one type of data may make conclusions far more robust, and thus a decision may be better delayed until further data are collected;
- decision-makers may use results from one type of sensitivity or scenario analysis dealing, for example, with a variable more in their control to set policy (e.g. setting the price of a drug);
- decision-makers in other settings (e.g. other countries) may also be able to draw alternative conclusions provided analysts have reported sufficiently detailed sensitivity analyses;
- estimates of the maximum willingness-to-pay by decision-makers for a unit of effect can be used to identify decisions. For example, $50 per DALY averted was adopted arbitrarily by the World Bank in 1993 as the threshold below which public-health interventions are deemed to be cost-effective in low-income settings.

Summary

You have learnt about identifying sources of uncertainty in cost-effectiveness estimates which fall into three broad areas: methodological; data requirements; and generalizability. You have seen how to perform a basic sensitivity analysis and how the results should be interpreted. In the next chapter you will learn about another way of testing the confidence of the results of economic evaluations.

References

Agro KE, Bradley CA, Mittmann N, Iskedjian M, Llerisch AL and Einarson TR (1997) Sensitivity analysis in health economics and pharmacoeconomic studies. *Pharmacoeconomics* 11(1):75–88.

Briggs A and Gray A (2000) Handling uncertainty when performing economic evaluation of healthcare interventions. *Health Technology Assessment* 3(2), www.hta.nhsweb.nhs.uk.

Gold MR, Siegel JE, Russell LB and Weinstein MC (eds) (1996) *Cost-effectiveness in health and medicine*. New York: Oxford University Press.

Hutubessy R, Chisholm D and Edejer TTT (2003) Generalised cost-effectiveness analysis for national-level priority-setting in the health sector. *Cost Effectiveness Analysis and Resource Allocation* 1:8.

Manning WG, Fryback DG and Weinstein MC (1996) Reflecting uncertainty in cost-effectiveness analysis, in MR Gold, JE Siegel, LB Russell and MC Weinstein (eds) *Cost-effectiveness in health and medicine*. New York: Oxford University Press.

Walker D and Fox-Rushby JA (2001) How to do (or not to do) . . . allowing for uncertainty in economic evaluations: sensitivity analysis. *Health Policy and Planning* 16(4):435–43.

15 Probabilistic sensitivity analysis

Overview

The importance of sensitivity analysis was emphasized in the previous chapter. Probabilistic sensitivity analysis (PSA) is similar to one-way and multi-way analysis in that it still involves exchanging original parameter values with different values. However, it requires specific attention because it differs significantly from basic sensitivity analysis. That said, it should be viewed as a complement to, rather than a replacement for, basic sensitivity analysis since PSA does not examine the impact of every type of uncertainty outlined in the previous chapter. In this chapter you will learn about the rationale for PSA, the principles of how it is undertaken and read a critique of it strengths and weaknesses.

Learning objectives

After working through this chapter, you will be able to:

- **explain what is meant by probabilistic sensitivity analysis**
- **understand its advantages compared with basic sensitivity analysis**
- **understand which variables should and shouldn't be entered into a PSA**
- **appreciate how the illustrated distributions are calculated**
- **understand how cost-effectiveness acceptability curves are constructed**
- **interpret results presented in the form of cost-effectiveness acceptability curves**
- **appreciate the potential contribution of value of information analysis**

Key terms

Monte Carlo simulation A type of modelling that uses random numbers to capture the effects of uncertainty.

Stochastic guess Pertaining to conjecture.

Value of information The monetary value attached to acquiring additional information.

What is the rationale for PSA?

It should be clear from reading the previous chapter that there are a number of limitations with (basic) one- and multi-way sensitivity analyses in the way that they estimate and express the uncertainty around an ICER. One advantage of PSA is that it demonstrates how the decision at hand changes given different willingnesses to pay for health improvements. Another advantage is that it considers the uncertainty surrounding all parameters *simultaneously*, rather than one or a few variables at a time.

This point can be illustrated by considering a very basic example. You saw in the previous chapter that variables are sometimes non-linear in terms of the way they are related to each other (perhaps they are multiplicative). If this is the case, two separate one-way sensitivity analyses will reveal the independent influence of the individual parameters on the ICER but will not reveal the joint impact of varying both variables. A simple solution to this problem would be to perform a multi-way sensitivity analysis and to vary both variables at once. However, there are two related problems with this approach. First, it is unlikely that an economic evaluation will contain only two variables. Second, it is very likely that third, fourth, fifth variables etc. would further contribute to the overall ICER in that they interact directly with variables one and two. The only real solution to this problem is, therefore, to consider the (joint) uncertainty surrounding all parameters at the same time.

How is a PSA performed?

A hypothetical example – an evaluation of drug treatment for people infected with HIV compared to a strategy of no drug treatment – will be used to illustrate how a PSA is performed. There are six steps to consider. You will need to:

- design and build a model structure;
- identify the stochastic parameters within the model;
- assign distributions to these and all other relevant parameters (four examples, A–D, will be illustrated in the text);
- run the analysis;
- plot the resulting ICER pairs on a graph;
- calculate and plot a cost-effectiveness acceptability curve.

Design and build a model structure

The first point to note is that PSA is used specifically in model-based economic evaluations. It is not used when the results from economic evaluations based on randomized trials (i.e. patient-level data) are being analysed. PSA does not require special consideration when designing a model structure, therefore the issues outlined in Chapters 4 and 5 are also applicable to models involving PSA.

Consider the model in Figure 15.1. Briefly, the rectangles indicate the discrete set of Markov health states. CD4 lymphocyte cell counts are a method of determining how well a person's immune system is functioning. Lower CD4 cell counts indicate a poorer functioning immune system compared to higher counts.

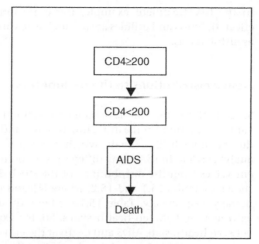

CD4 = lymphocyte cell count

Figure 15.1 A simple model of progression from healthy to dead
Source: Chancellor *et al.* (1997)

All patients enter the model in the healthiest state, CD4≥200 cells μ/L. The arrows indicate the possible transitions (as you learned in Chapter 5, known as transition probabilities) between health states as well as the direction of travel, although the model also allows people to remain in the same health state. The purpose of treatment is to slow the rate at which CD4 counts decline and ultimately to slow the rate at which people progress to AIDS (an indication of a severely compromised immune system) and death. The model cycles annually for ten years. Deaths from non-HIV/AIDS related causes are not included in this example.

Identify the stochastic parameters within the model

PSA considers the uncertainty around the value of a parameter (this is known as second-order uncertainty). It does this by specifying relevant parameters as distributions rather than point estimates. It does not consider uncertainty in the variability of an underlying population from which the sample is drawn (first-order uncertainty). Nor does it consider methodological or other types of uncertainty.

Given this, it is important that you understand which variables in a model should be specified as distributions and which should not. Consider the following example. The effects of providing mosquito nets could be a function of whether they are used correctly and whether they are well maintained. Both of these variables are arguably measurable and, as such, are stochastic (a guess) and will have an associated variance. Thus they can be fitted with a distribution. However, variables such as the rates at which costs and benefits are discounted are determined by you (albeit often with advice from third parties) and do not vary within a simulation. Another example of a variable that is typically non-stochastic is the time horizon of the analysis.

In the HIV treatment example, the transition probabilities, relative treatment effect, the costs and utilities are all stochastic variables and thus should be specified as distributions.

Assign distributions to the parameters

So far in this book, you have seen that ICERs are estimated by combining all relevant information on mean treatment costs and mean effects. This approach produces a single ICER estimate, which is sometimes referred to as a deterministic (or analytic) ICER. In PSA many different ICER points are generated by drawing different values from the distributions of the stochastic variables. Consider the values shown in Tables 15.1 and 15.2, where NT and DT refer to 'no therapy' and 'drug therapy' respectively. Table 15.1 contains the transition probabilities associated with moving between health states. So, for example, the probability of moving between health state AIDS and death at the end of a year is 0.6 for people receiving no therapy. Table 15.2 contains the costs and utilities associated with each of these health states for both the NT and DT options. Note that the drug therapy is assumed to have no associated adverse effects, thus the utilities for NT and DT are identical.

Table 15.1 Deterministic transition matrix for baseline risk of disease progression for no therapy

From state:	CD4≥200 cells m/L	To state: CD4<200 cells m/L	AIDS	Death
CD4≥200 cells m/L	(1−0.5)	0.5	–	–
CD4<200 cells m/L	–	(1−0.4)	0.4	–
AIDS	–	–	(1−0.6)	0.6

Table 15.2 Deterministic health state mean costs (£) and utilities

	CD4≥200 cells m/L	CD4<200 cells m/L	AIDS	Death
Costs$_{NT}$	50	100	200	0
Cost$_{DT}$	100	150	250	0
Utility$_{NT}$	0.82	0.79	0.5	0
Utility$_{DT}$	0.82	0.79	0.5	0

At the moment, the transition probabilities, costs and utilities are all specified as point estimates. The next step is to turn them into distributions. The important point to note is that the appropriate distribution to use depends on the type of variable that is under consideration; the choice of appropriate distribution is not arbitrary. Typically, the parameters used to specify these distributions are derived from the literature (as is the case for all parameters in model-based economic evaluations!).

Probabilities

Probabilities have a number of properties – most importantly they are a continuous distribution and bounded between 0 and 1 (that is, their value cannot be below 0 or above 1). Because of this, beta distributions are a natural choice to assign to probabilities. A beta distribution has the following functional form Be ~ (alpha, beta), where alpha is the number of observed events in a given time period and beta is the sample size minus alpha.

Assume that for the health state CD4<200 cells μ/L, 40 (alpha) out of 100 people progress to AIDS at the end of each cycle; hence a probability of (40/100) 0.4 is specified in the relevant cell in the deterministic transition matrix. However, the appropriate parameters, when specified as a beta distribution are, in this example, Be ~ (40, 60). These are the numbers that should be entered into the model instead of the original 0.5 (see Figure 15.2). This should be repeated for all the probabilities in the transition matrix. There is no need to assign beta distributions to the remaining cells because they are either 0 or can be calculated from another cell that has already been assigned a distribution.

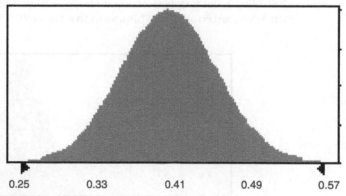

0.25   0.33   0.41   0.49   0.57

Figure 15.2 Beta distribution with alpha = 40 and beta = 60

Relative risks

This model also includes a relative risk of disease progression, which represents the treatment effect of using a drug therapy relative to no treatment. Relative risks are typically specified as log-normal distributions because of their ratio properties.

Assume that the relative risk of disease progression is 0.9 (95% CI 0.81–0.99). A log-normal distribution has the following functional form Ln ~ (mean, sd). In this example, Ln ~ (–0.105, 0.05) following standard statistical principles. Remember that the generated results will be on the log-normal scale, thus will need to be exponentiated following the simulation (see Figure 15.3).

Costs

Cost data cannot be negative thus values are either zero or positive. Because of this, they are typically specified as either gamma or log-normal distributions.

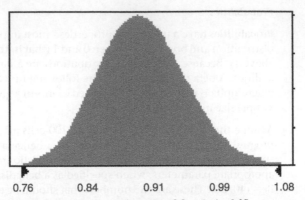

0.76	0.84	0.91	0.99	1.08

Figure 15.3 Log-normal distribution with mean = 0.9 and sd = 0.05

A gamma distribution is specified as Ga ~ (alpha, beta). Where alpha equals the mean cost squared divided by the standard deviation squared and beta equals the standard deviation squared divided by the mean cost. Assume for health state CD4≥ ≥200 cells μ/L (for people receiving no treatment) that the annual mean cost is £50 with a standard error of £6. This means that Ga ~ (69, 0.7) (see Figure 15.4).

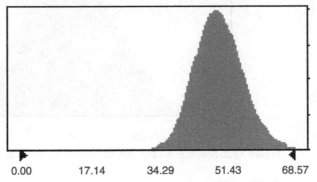

0.00	17.14	34.29	51.43	68.57

Figure 15.4 Gamma distribution with alpha = 69 and beta = 0.7

Utilities

Utilities cannot have a value greater than 1 but are not bounded by 0 as health states ranked worse than death are possible. Adjustments to accommodate negative values exist. However, when values are positive and far from 0, the pragmatic approach is to fit a beta distribution.

Utility data are often reported as means and standard deviations. Consider the value assigned to health state Utility$_{NT}$ of 0.82 and assume this has a standard deviation of 0.08, this produces Be ~ (19, 4). Where alpha equals the mean squared multiplied by 1 minus the mean and beta equals alpha divided by the mean minus alpha.

Run the analysis

Once the model has been populated with the relevant data, a number of simulations should be run (say 10,000). The purpose of running the model more than once is to allow sampling from the various distributions. For each simulation, different values will be picked from the distributions, thus many different ICERs will be calculated. Another way to think about this is that there would be little point in specifying a variable as a distribution and then only sampling from it once. Simulations are often performed using a technique known as 'Monte Carlo simulation' analysis – a method commonly used to sample randomly from distributions. The result, in this instance is 10,000 ICER pairs, with a mean ICER of approximately £780 per additional QALY.

Plot the resulting ICER pairs on a graph

The results from a simulation can be plotted on a cost-effectiveness plane (see Figure 15.5). The illustration shows that on the vast majority of occasions, the drug was more costly and more effective than not treating patients – hence most of the plots are in the NE quadrant of the plane. However, it also shows that on a small number of occasions, drug treatment was both more costly and less effective compared with no treatment and vice versa.

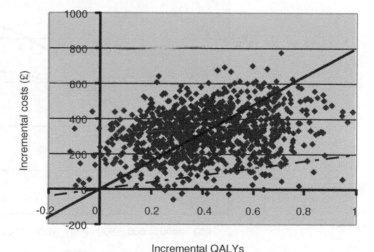

Figure 15.5 Cost-effectiveness plane

Calculate and plot a cost-effectiveness acceptability curve

The next step is to plot a cost-effectiveness acceptability curve. The curve is useful for at least two reasons. First, it shows how the decision to adopt a technology changes as the threshold value of health gain changes. This is useful because in practice this value is not known (at least not with any degree of accuracy). Second, the curve provides a means of combining information on the uncertainties associated with the variables. Also it avoids the need to calculate confidence intervals (and some inherent statistical problems).

To understand how the curve is calculated, return to Figure 15.5. The dashed and solid lines indicate maximum willingness to pay thresholds of £200 and £800 per additional QALY respectively. The curve is constructed by counting the number of ICERs that fall below these values and by plotting the results. This is repeated for all threshold values of interest to build up the curve, starting at 0 and increasing to a maximum threshold value of choice (in this instance, £2000).

The acceptability curve is shown in Figure 15.6 (solid line). It is clear from the curve that as the threshold value for an ICER increases, so does the probability that drug therapy is the more cost-effective option. However, at values of (say) £500, drug therapy was only considered to be cost-effective on approximately 20% of occasions compared to no therapy, and therefore would not represent value for money at this threshold value. Also note in this example that at no point is drug therapy associated with a 100% probability of being cost-effective. This is because there are a number of simulations that suggest it produces fewer QALYs at greater cost compared with no therapy. Note that the mean ICER is found at a willingness to pay threshold of approximately 50%.

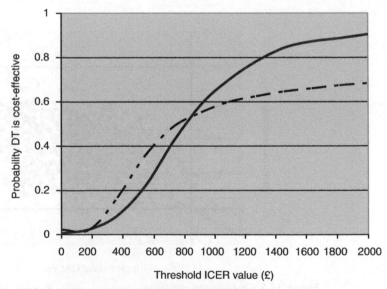

Figure 15.6 Cost-effectiveness acceptability curve (CEAC)

The dashed line shows what happens to the curve when the uncertainty around the relative risk is increased (but not the mean value). Most notably, the curve (CEAC) clearly shows that less certainty is attached to higher threshold WTP values. Note also that the dashed line intersects the y-axis above 0 (although only just above 0). This is because on a small but non-negligible number of occasions, drug therapy was shown to be more effective and less costly than no therapy. Therefore, even if the WTP for an extra unit of health was 0, drug therapy was cost-effective on a small number of occasions.

 Activity 15.1

Consider an intervention which can be characterized by the combinations of incremental cost and incremental effectiveness shown in the cost-effectiveness plane in Figure 15.7, where the two ellipses contain 50 and 95% of the points. Note that while most of the points are in the NE quadrant there are (ΔE, ΔC) combinations in all of the other quadrants. Draw the cost-effectiveness acceptability curve associated with this intervention and explain why it has this shape and position.

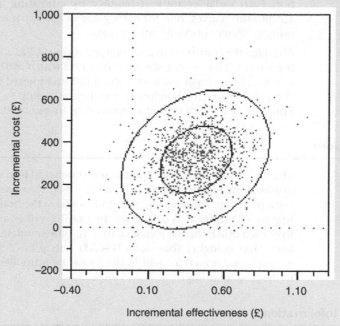

Figure 15.7 Cost-effectiveness plane including 50 and 95% confidence ellipses

 Feedback

With a zero value attached to the additional QALYs the intervention will be cost-effective in those cases where it is cost-saving. As the value per additional QALY increases there will be an increasing number of combinations of (ΔE, ΔC) where the intervention is cost-effective. However, no matter how high a value is placed on additional QALYs there will remain combinations of (ΔE, ΔC) where the intervention is not cost-effective. Thus the cost-effectiveness curve will start at a positive value (slightly greater than zero) and will rise levelling off at a value below 1.

Comparing three or more options

The example has considered the case of two options where the results can be summarized by a single cost-effectiveness acceptability curve. When there are three or more options a cost-effectiveness acceptability curve can be drawn for each one, each curve showing the probability that that option is the most cost-effective for each particular monetary value of the outcome. The probabilities of each option being cost-effective at each monetary value should always sum to 1.

Non-sampling uncertainty

Clearly while sampling variation is an important source of uncertainty, as noted in Chapter 14, it is not the only source of uncertainty. Instead of specifying a distribution, such variables are best handled by estimating multiple cost-effectiveness acceptability curves, one for each value of the variable of interest. For example, using a different discount rate for costs.

Although the construction and interpretation of CEACs should be clear, sometimes the mean ICER does not always correspond with a 50% probability of being cost-effective. This happens when the distributions inputted into the model are skewed. When this happens therefore, it can be misleading to simply rely on the curve. Thus, the mean ICER should also always be investigated.

Correlations

The standard approach to Monte Carlo simulation is to sample randomly from the distributions independently from each other. However, this 'independence' can cause problems. For example, the utility value in the health state AIDS is lower than that for CD4<200 cells μ/L. If the two utility values are sampled independently from each other, there is a chance that in some simulations utility value associated with AIDS is higher than for CD4<200 cells μ/L. Clearly this isn't correct and should be accounted for within the model by introducing correlation coefficients to the programming.

Value of information

Value of information (VOI) is a type of analysis that can be performed using the results from a PSA. The question often arises whether it is worth spending extra resources reducing the uncertainty around an ICER before making a decision; or which research activities should be the priority given that research funds are scarce.

VOI is useful because it helps to answer these questions. More specifically, it provides an analytical framework which can be used to quantify the maximum societal value of additional investigation. In so doing, it helps to bring focus to research activities where more information would be most valuable. 'Information is valuable because it reduces the expected costs of uncertainty surrounding a clinical decision. The expected costs of uncertainty can also be interpreted as the expected value of perfect information (EVPI) since perfect information (an infinite sample) can eliminate the possibility of making the wrong decision' (Claxton 1999).

EVPI is calculated by subtracting the expected value of current information from the expected value of having perfect information. An example of perfect information could be a test for a disease that is 100% accurate. The calculation also formally takes into account the willingness to pay for an extra unit of health and the number of people who are likely to benefit from the extra research (since research is considered to be a public good). If the cost of acquiring further information is greater than the EVPI, then further research is not worthwhile on economic grounds.

In order to determine whether it is worth collecting additional information (and the extent and form this should take) it is necessary to consider the expected value of sample information (EVSI) relative to its cost. For example, larger samples will be expected to produce better information and so the EVSI rises. But larger samples will increase the cost of acquiring this information. In deciding on the sample size the increased benefit must be set against the increased cost. This is done by maximizing the expected net benefit of sampling (ENBS). This is the difference between the EVSI and the cost of acquiring this information. All research will have some fixed costs (regardless of the sample size) and for it to be worthwhile undertaking the research the ENBS must exceed these fixed costs.

Consider the following example adapted from Claxton (1999). It features an intervention where the current estimate of incremental cost is $5000 and incremental benefit is 0.2 QALYs giving an ICER of $25,000 per QALY. It highlights that the ENBS depends on:

- the prior information available;
- the marginal cost of sampling;
- the size of the patient population (who could benefit).

Table 15.3 presents four of the possible combinations of these factors and also considers two different monetary valuations of a QALY.

Table 15.3 Four combinations of prior information, marginal cost of sampling and size of patient population

	Case 1: good prior information; high marginal sampling cost; small patient population	Case 2: good prior information; low marginal sampling cost; small patient population	Case 3: poor prior information; low marginal sampling cost; small patient population	Case 4: poor prior information; low marginal sampling cost; large patient population
EVPI				
value of QALY $30,000	$9.2 m	$9.2 m	$16.4 m	$81.8 m
value of a QALY $50,000	$9.8 m	$9.8 m	$21.0 m	$104.8 m
Optimal sample size				
value of QALY $30,000	398	508	580	1754
value of a QALY $50,000	0	609	744	2129
Maximum ENBS				
value of QALY $30,000	$1.2 m	$1.6 m	$7.6 m	$58.0 m
value of a QALY $50,000	$0 m	$0.3 m	$8.9 m	$72.0 m

Source: Adapted from Claxton (1999)

Activity 15.2

Considering Table 15.3:

1 Why is the EVPI highest in Case 4 where the value of a QALY is $50,000?
2 What does a maximum ENBS of zero imply about future research?
3 Why might the value of a QALY affect Cases 2 and 3 differently?

Feedback

1 The returns from investing in further information are greater when the health benefits are valued more highly, where initial information is poorer and the costs of acquiring better information are lower.

2 Additional research is of low value relative to its cost.

3 The value of a QALY has a bigger effect when initial information is poorer and there is more to learn.

Activity 15.3

Given the factors which influence the efficiency of additional research highlighted in Table 15.3, identify two examples of research which are likely to have a low ENBS and two examples of research which would have a high ENBS.

Feedback

Your low ENBS examples are likely to feature conditions where a large amount is known, and the treatments have been evaluated in several randomized trials with suitably large sample sizes and durations of follow-up. It is likely that there has been good agreement across the results of the trials. The potential population of patients who could benefit is probably not large and it may be that the marginal sampling cost is high. In contrast, the examples of high ENBS will probably involve a larger number of potential beneficiaries, a less well-researched treatment (possibly because it is a new technology) and a lower marginal sampling cost (possibly shorter follow-up study is required, or lower costs of identifying suitable patients).

Summary

You have learnt about PSA, an approach that complements basic sensitivity analysis. You have seen when it is appropriate to use it, how it is undertaken and its strengths and weaknesses.

References

Chancellor JV, Hill AM, Sabin CA, Simpson KN and Youle M (1997) Modelling the cost effectiveness of lamivudine/zidovudine combination therapy in HIV infection. *Pharmaco-Economics* 12:54–66.

Claxton K (1999) Bayesian approaches to the value of information: implications for the regulation of new pharmaceuticals. *Health Economics* 8:269–74.

Further reading

Fenwick E, O'Brien BJ and Briggs A (2004) Cost-effectiveness acceptability curves – facts, fallacies and frequently asked questions. *Health Economics* 13:405–15.

16 Guidelines for economic evaluation

Overview

Guidelines for economic evaluation of health care interventions have been around for more than 30 years but have changed over time. Initially they were largely instructive, aimed at encouraging wider use of economic methods in a field where decision-making often ignored economic issues. As interest grew and there were many new entrants to the health economic arena they became more concerned with encouraging good practice. More recently the driver for guideline development has been the growing need to provide and assess evidence of cost-effectiveness for reimbursement purposes. Bodies requiring such evidence encourage the development and use of guidelines as a means of assisting their decision-making.

Learning objectives

After working through this chapter, you will be able to:

- discuss the potential advantages and disadvantages of guidelines for economic evaluation
- understand the nature and relevance of a reference case
- outline the methods required by economic evaluations produced to inform the appraisal of health technologies in England and Wales

Key terms

Reference case A set of assumptions and methods, which should wherever possible be followed by all economic evaluations so that different studies can be more readily compared.

Introduction

It would be difficult to make a convincing case against having any guidelines whatsoever with respect to economic evaluation. In any case, on a more pragmatic note, guidelines exist and are not going to go away. Rather, the issues are how important are they, what efforts should be invested in developing and implementing them, and how should they be used in order to enhance the contribution of economic evaluation to health care decision-making?

Guidelines for economic evaluation

Guidelines have been developed for the conduct and reporting of economic evaluations. They come in a number of different forms, ranging from formal guidelines which must be followed when presenting evidence on cost-effectiveness to a body with responsibility for making reimbursement decisions, to the informal – essentially suggestions of good practice which may only be written with respect to particular aspects of evaluation, for example costing or estimating WTP. The focus in this chapter is on the more formal end of this spectrum. Such guidelines seek to improve the quality of economic evaluations by encouraging (or requiring) good practice. They also lead to greater standardization of studies which in turn increases the comparability of studies and, possibly, the generalizability of results. Assessment of cost-effectiveness evidence is facilitated by reducing the heterogeneity of evaluations.

As governments around the world have increasingly recognized a need for research evidence, not just on the safety and efficacy of new interventions but also on cost-effectiveness, interest in guidelines for economic evaluation has grown considerably. As a result guidelines exist for many high-income countries. Hjelmgren *et al.* (2001) review 25 guidelines issued in Europe, North America and Australasia. The initial emphasis on formulating guidelines for low- and middle-income countries focused on guidelines for specific disease programmes (Walker 2001). More recently WHO have produced guidelines on generalized cost-effectiveness analysis (Tan-Torres Edejer *et al.* 2003).

Advantages and disadvantages of guidelines

Guidelines are valuable in a number of ways. First, they encourage you to be more explicit because they require clear statements of, and sometimes justifications for, the choices you make. Second, and partly as a result of increased explicitness, they increase comparability of studies. Third, more speculatively, they may bring benefits in terms of quality control. Thus at first sight they appear to be a quite reasonable notion. Few would argue against the desirability of explicitness, greater comparability and improvements in the quality of evaluations.

However, there are a number of reasons why guidelines (or more precisely continuing efforts to develop guidelines) should not be welcomed uncritically. First, guidelines presuppose a fairly large measure of consensus over methods, whereas there are many issues over which there is not yet agreement. Some of these have their root in ideological differences that cannot be expected to be resolved but some also stem from a basic lack of knowledge (or possibly a failure to assimilate the available information). Second, the development of guidelines as with any other activity has an opportunity cost and it is appropriate to ask how the incremental benefit from further development of guidelines compares with the incremental cost. One of the more subtle elements of opportunity cost might be the discouragement of research. If particular methodological practices become enshrined in a guideline it may become harder to obtain funding to study other approaches and harder to publish research based on methods not approved by the ruling guidelines. The discouragement of research could then become institutionalized and innovation may be discouraged.

The opportunity cost of the development of guidelines for economic evaluation is a theme developed by Maynard (1997): 'Investment in the improvement of guidelines and development of consensus about best practice yields a small marginal product'. One problem he highlights is the way in which the development of guidelines diverts attention away from unresolved issues. Instead of seeking to refine guidelines, efforts might give a greater return by monitoring the *practice* of economic evaluation. A number of studies which have reviewed the conduct of economic evaluation have reached similar conclusions regarding the small proportion that attain the highest standards (Udvarhelyi *et al.* 1992). Indeed, dissatisfaction over the standards of economic evaluation has been one of the engines which drives interest in guidelines. However, it is clearly not the lack of guidelines which is responsible for low-quality evaluations in that guidelines have been available for years. Thus if the quality of many evaluations is a major concern, the preferred policy for raising standards is unlikely to involve the further development of guidelines but rather needs to consider why, when guidelines have existed for such a long time, they have so little impact.

If guidelines don't change practice, the fears about the deleterious impact on research are possibly unfounded, but concern that the development and refinement of guidelines is not a good use of scarce resources will grow.

At least one prominent health economist has voiced concern that some of the interest in the development and use of guidelines is driven by commercial rather than scientific motives (Evans 1995). In short, guidelines may be of potential benefit to the pharmaceutical industry but are they of potential benefit to a wider community?

Whatever view is taken on their desirability, guidelines are clearly here to stay. You will now turn to an important vehicle by which guidelines are influencing the conduct of evaluation – the reference case.

 Activity 16.1

To what extent is there a danger that guidelines for economic evaluation of health care, in attempting to encourage good practice, might discourage good research?

 Feedback

Clearly different answers to this question are possible. Your answer should consider what is good practice and what is good research. It should also recognize that there are arguments both for and against the position. To what extent is this a researchable question rather than an act of faith?

Reference case concept

In 1993 the US Public Health Service convened a Panel on Cost-Effectiveness in Health and Medicine (known as the Washington Panel) (Gold *et al.* 1996). The Panel wished to increase comparability of cost-effectiveness analyses while still permitting analysts sufficient flexibility to undertake evaluations appropriate to their specific circumstances. They identified the use of a reference case as a means of achieving these twin goals. For the Panel, 'the reference case is a standard set of methodologic practices that an analyst would seek to follow in a cost-effectiveness study'. Analysts might well also choose to use different assumptions and methods but the reference case would be a common feature across studies, thus enabling different studies to be readily compared. The Panel recognized that cost-effectiveness analyses ranged widely in scope and purpose and thus comparability wrought through the reference case would not always be a primary concern. However, for a growing number of studies on the cost-effectiveness of health care interventions, comparability with other studies was a central concern and thus analysts would want to feature the reference case.

NICE guidance on methods

NICE, among other activities, produces guidance on the use of new and existing interventions within the NHS in England and Wales. In reaching its judgement it is required to have regard to:

- broad clinical priorities;
- the degree of clinical need;
- the broad balance of benefits and costs;
- any guidance on the resources likely to be available; and
- the effective use of available resources.

These wider concerns have been operationalized as the assessment of clinical and cost-effectiveness. Submissions from manufacturers or sponsors of health technologies and from an independent academic assessment group are important inputs to NICE's decision-making. To facilitate review of this evidence NICE has embraced the concept of a reference case. Submissions can depart from the reference case but these departures must be justified. Note this is a slightly more prescriptive approach than originally envisioned by the Washington Panel.

NICE's primary concern is to adopt a consistent approach when appraising clinical and cost-effectiveness across different interventions and disease areas (NICE 2004). While it is recognized that there is debate about the most appropriate methods to be used for some aspects of health technology assessment, the reference case specifies the methods believed to be the most appropriate for informing decisions and is consistent with the objective of maximizing health gain from available resources.

It is explicitly recognized that data required to present reference case results are not always available (this is frequently the case with respect to the measurement of quality of life). But it is emphasized that in such cases any departures from the reference case should be clearly specified and justified. Indeed, the likely implications of departing from the reference case have to be quantified.

The main elements of the NICE reference case are summarized in Table 16.1. While much of the reference case is quite unremarkable there are a number of ways in which this guide is distinctive. First, the firm endorsement of probabilistic sensitivity analysis to handle parameter uncertainty. Second, the requirement for QALYs to be based on a standardized and validated generic instrument and for the

Table 16.1 The NICE reference case

Element of health technology assessment	Reference case
Defining the decision problem	The scope is developed by NICE prior to the independent academic assessment
Comparator	Alternative therapies routinely used in the NHS
Perspective on costs	NHS and personal social services
Perspective on outcomes	All health effects on individuals
Type of economic evaluation	CEA
Synthesis of evidence on outcomes	Based on a systematic review
Measure of health benefits	QALYs
Description of health states for calculation of QALYs	Health states described using a standardized and validated generic instrument
Method of preference elicitation for health state valuation	Choice-based method, for example, TTO, SG (not rating scale)
Source of preference data	Representative sample of the (UK) public
Modelling methods	Models used to synthesize evidence should follow accepted guidelines. Full documentation and justification of structural assumptions and data inputs should be provided
Time horizon	Sufficiently long to reflect any differences in costs or outcomes between the technologies being compared
Discount rate	An annual rate of 3.5% on both costs and health effects
Treatment of uncertainty	PSA should be used to translate the imprecision in all input variables into a measure of decision uncertainty. Sensitivity analysis should be used to deal with sources of uncertainty other than that related to the precision of the parameter estimates
Reporting cost-effectiveness	Present expected value of each component of cost, expected total costs and expected QALYs for each option. ICERs should be calculated as appropriate
Sub-group analysis	Separate estimates of clinical and cost effectiveness should be made for each sub-group where capacity to benefit from treatment differs
Equity position	An additional QALY has the same weight regardless of the other characteristics of the individuals receiving the health benefit

Source: NICE (2004)

preferences of the UK general public to be elicited using a choice-based method comes close to requesting that the EQ5D be used.

 Activity 16.2

Review the different elements of health technology appraisal listed in Table 16.1. Which of these contribute most to facilitating comparison of different studies? Which of these elements are unnecessary or less important for facilitating comparability of studies?

Feedback

Which elements contribute most and which are less important could depend on the specific study. For example, the discount rate may frequently not be very important but in certain circumstances it can be very important. If studies measure the same costs and health benefits in similar terms this would assist comparison. Similarly, the time horizon and the reporting of results are likely to be important, whereas exactly *how* uncertainty has been handled may be less important.

Summary

You have learnt about the potential advantages and disadvantages of imposing guidelines on how to undertake economic evaluations. You went on to see how in one particular country the central government was making use of economic evaluations in decision-making.

References

Evans RG (1995) Manufacturing consensus, marketing truth: guidelines for economic evaluation. *Annals of Internal Medicine* 123:59–60.

Gold MR, Siegel JE, Russell LB and Weinstein MC (eds) (1996) *Cost-effectiveness in health and medicine.* Oxford: Oxford University Press.

Hjelmgren J, Berggren F and Andersson F (2001) Health economic guidelines – similarities, differences and some implications. *Value Health* 4:225–50.

Maynard A (1997) Economic evaluation techniques in healthcare: reinventing the wheel? *PharmacoEconomics* 11:115–18.

NICE (2004) *Guide to the methods of technology appraisal.* London: NICE, www.nice.org.uk.

Tan-Torres Edejer T *et al.* (eds) *Making choices in health: WHO guide to cost-effectiveness analysis.* Geneva: WHO, www.who.int.

Udvarhelyi IS, Colditz GA, Rai A and Epstein AM (1992) Cost-effectiveness and cost-benefit analysis in the medical literature: are methods being used correctly? *Annals of Internal Medicine* 116:238–44.

Walker D (2001) Cost and cost-effectiveness guidelines: which ones to use? *Health Policy and Planning* 16:113–21.

Further reading

www.ispor.org/PEguidelines/index.asp.

SECTION 5

Appraising the quality and usefulness of economic evaluation

17 | Critical appraisal of an economic evaluation

Overview

This chapter provides a means by which you can assess the quality and relevance of an economic evaluation. A series of questions are identified which you should ask of any economic evaluation. In principle, this should allow you to determine the quality of the economic evaluation and thus, to some extent, the weight it should be given with respect to informing decision-making. The transferability (or otherwise) of results is taken up in the next chapter.

Learning objectives

After working through this chapter, you will be able to:

- **list the important questions to ask in order to assess the quality of an economic evaluation**
- **understand why the answers to these questions are informative**
- **undertake a critical appraisal of an economic evaluation**

Introduction

The number of economic evaluations published increases year on year. This is good news for those looking for information with which to inform decision-making regarding the allocation of resources in health care. But it brings with it a number of challenges – for example, determining which studies to give greater weight when not all studies reach the same conclusion.

The rapid pace of expansion of evaluation has had a number of consequences – several studies may be available of any particular intervention and a large number of researchers have become involved from a wide variety of backgrounds. There has also been rapid technological advance in the conduct of economic evaluation. While this must be welcomed, it brings additional challenges in assessing the quality of evaluations. Also, evaluations are becoming more complex and thus are making greater demands on the expertise of the users of the information generated.

This expansion of activity has increased interest in guidelines for the conduct and reporting of studies. This is illustrated in this chapter by the move from simple checklists of questions to much more detailed and specific questions being asked of studies.

Table 17.1 reproduces the abbreviated list of questions suggested by Mike Drummond when assessing the quality of an economic evaluation. While this serves as an excellent starting point, a rather more detailed set of questions is required to provide insight into the specific shortcomings of a study. Such a list is provided by the *British Medical Journal* (Drummond and Jefferson 1996). The latter has been devised for a specific purpose, namely to inform decisions whether or not to publish a study. Thus it is particularly concerned with the quality of the reporting of a study and is less prescriptive about the conduct of the evaluation. However, it provides a sharper focus than the earlier Drummond checklist.

Table 17.1 The Drummond Checklist

Q1	Well-defined question?
Q2	Description of alternatives?
Q3	Effectiveness established?
Q4	All relevant costs and consequences?
Q5	Appropriate measurement?
Q6	Credible valuation?
Q7	Differential timing?
Q8	Incremental costs and consequences?
Q9	Allowance made for uncertainty?
Q10	Appropriate interpretation of results?

Source: Adapted from Drummond et al. (1987)

These guidelines can be arranged in three groups: study design; data collection; and analysis and interpretation of results. Clearly not all items are of equal importance and the relative importance of different items is not fixed but will depend on the purpose of the study. Having worked through this book you will have already encountered discussion on most of the elements identified.

Study design

The items with respect to study design are concerned with whether or not the approach adopted is clearly stated and to a lesser extent with whether or not it has been justified. This initial set of items fairly clearly reflects the needs of the readers of a journal. For example, whether the economic importance of the research question is stated is hardly much of a guide to the quality of the evaluation, but a general reader in allocating their time or an editor in allocating space may prefer questions of economic importance. Whether the form of economic evaluation used is stated again hardly reflects on the quality of the evaluation. The form will be self-evident on reading but for the busy reader it is more convenient to be told.

Of much greater importance to any users of the analysis are whether or not the options being compared have been clearly described and that the case has been made that these are the appropriate comparisons to make.

Data collection

The set of items relating to the effectiveness of the interventions are of particular importance. Without detailed information on the sources of information and the methods used it is impossible for the reader to know what credence to give the results.

The items provide a major challenge to an author writing a journal article particularly if, as is increasingly the case, a model is used in the study. As models have become more widely used and usually more complex, a stage has been reached where even a fairly detailed description of the model may not provide enough information for it to be adequately assessed. At least a detailed description of the model may provide the reader with some reassurance regarding the quality and relevance of the study.

Some items, such as reporting quantities of resources separately from their unit costs, and details of currency conversions and price bases, are fairly straightforward to implement. As you will see in the next chapter, these are important as regards the transferability of results.

Analysis and interpretation of results

The issues are listed in Table 17.2. The items with respect to the time horizon and the discounting of costs and effects belong in the easily implemented category. The standard of reporting with respect to these items, particularly in recent years, is generally fairly high.

Table 17.2 Analysis and interpretation items

- Time horizon of costs and benefits is stated
- The discount rate(s) is stated and justified and an explanation is given if costs or benefits are not discounted
- Details of statistical tests and confidence intervals are given for stochastic data
- The approach to sensitivity analysis is given and the choice of variables for sensitivity analysis and the ranges over which the variables are varied are justified
- Relevant alternatives are compared
- Incremental analysis is reported
- Major outcomes are presented in a disaggregated as well as aggregated form
- The answer to the study question is given
- Conclusions follow from the data reported and are accompanied by the appropriate caveats

Source: Adapted from Drummond and Jefferson (1996)

Transparency with respect to sensitivity analysis is particularly important. As emphasized in Chapters 14 and 15 all evaluations are characterized by substantial uncertainties and it is very important that these are appropriately explored in any analysis. Sensitivity analysis has been an area where practice has often lagged behind the methods available. Also the value of the additional insights that can be derived from a well-conducted and reported sensitivity analysis is substantial.

Whether the answer to the study question is given and whether the conclusions follow from the data reported is concerned with good practice for the convenience to journal readers. While a careful reading of a paper will reveal whether it has succeeded in answering the study question and whether the conclusions follow the analysis, failure with respect to these items is not overly serious. However, there is a real danger of misleading some readers if these good practices are not observed.

Activity 17.1

Suppose you are a health care purchaser who has responsibility for the acute care budget for your local population.

1 Which items would you regard as essential?
2 Which would you regard as desirable but not essential?
3 Is there any other information that would assist you in deciding whether or not a particular study could inform your decision-making?

 Feedback

1 The items that you have identified as essential would be likely to include most if not all of the following: the research question is stated; the viewpoint(s) of the analysis are clearly stated and justified; the alternatives being compared are clearly described; the source(s) of effectiveness estimates used are stated; the primary outcome measure for the economic evaluation is clearly stated; quantities of resources are reported separately from their unit costs; methods for the estimation of quantities and unit costs are described; currency and price data are recorded; the choice of model used and the key parameters on which it is based are justified; the time horizon of costs and benefits is stated; the choice of variables for sensitivity analysis is justified; incremental analysis is reported; and conclusions follow from the data reported.

2 Details of the design and results of the effectiveness study, of the method of data synthesis, of the methods to value health states, and of the subjects. Also the range over which variables are varied, disaggregated major outcomes, and conclusions accompanied by the appropriate caveats.

3 Explicit discussion of transferability and details of any potential conflicts of interest.

 Activity 17.2

Dzeikan et al. (2003) model the cost-effectiveness of policies for the safe and appropriate use of injections in ten regions of the world. Write a review of their paper, an abridged version of which appears below. You need to consider the items that have been discussed.

 The cost-effectiveness of policies for injection use

Methods

The six regions of WHO were separated into subgroups of countries on the basis of having similar rates of child and adult mortality. This resulted in 14 Global Burden of Disease 2000 epidemiological subregions characterized by the WHO region acronyms (AFR (African Region); AMR (Region of the Americas); EMR (Eastern Mediterranean Region); EUR (European Region); SEAR (South-East Asia Region); and WPR (Western Pacific Region)) and a letter for the mortality stratum (Table 17.3).

Table 17.3 Contaminated injections burden of disease

	African region		Region of the Americas		Eastern Mediterranean	European region		South-East Asia region		Western Pacific
	AFR D	AFR E	AMR B	AMR D	EMR D	EUR B	EUR C	SEAR B	SEAR D	WPR B
Mortality in children	High	High	Low	High	High	Low	Low	Low	High	Low
Mortality in adults	High	Very high	Low	High	High	Low	Low	Low	High	Low
Injections per person per year[1]	2.2	2.0	1.7	1.9	4.3	5.2	11.3	2.1	4.0	2.4
Proportion of reuse (%)[1]	19	17	1.2	11	70	1.2	11	30	75	30
Total Burden 2000–30[1]	555 644	1 668 583	9 083	27 332	559 702	3 479	64 733	280 789	4 720 866	1 287 470
Preventable burden 2000–33										
Reduction of injection use[2]	166 193	500 575	2 725	8 200	167 911	1 044	19 420	84 237	1 416 260	386 241
Reduction of unsafe use[3]	527 862	1 585 154	8 629	25 965	531 717	3 305	61 496	266 749	4 484 823	1 223 096
Combined interventions	536 197	1 610 182	8 765	26 375	540 112	3 357	62 467	270 961	4 555 636	1 242 408

1 'Do nothing' scenario
2 Interactional group discussions between patients and providers to reduce injection use
3 Provision of single use, disposable syringes and needles for all injections
Source: Dziekan et al. (2003)

Effectiveness model

We considered a theoretical cohort of the population living in the year 2000 in subregions where reuse of injection equipment has been reported. We first applied a current, 'do nothing' scenario where persons were injected using contaminated needles and consequently acquired infections. Second, we applied a series of hypothetical intervention scenarios for the year 2000, taking into account the effect of these interventions on the incidence of infections.

DALYs attributable to poor injection practices

We modelled the fraction of incident HBV, HCV, and HIV infections attributable to contaminated injections on the basis of the annual number of injections per person, the proportion of injections administered with equipment reused in the absence of sterilization, the probability of transmission following percutaneous exposure, the prevalence of active infection, the prevalence of immunity, and the incidence. The burden in DALYs for the years 2000–30 due to infections in the year 2000 was estimated on the basis of the natural history of viral infections, background mortality, Global Burden of Disease life tables, and the average duration and disability weights of acute hepatitis, cirrhosis, hepatocellular carcinoma, and AIDS. DALYs were age-weighted and 3% discounted.

Effectiveness of interventions

We examined interventions for reducing the unsafe use of injections, interventions for reducing injection use, and the effect of these two interventions when implemented jointly. For interventions to reduce the unsafe use of injections, we considered the effectiveness of interventions on the basis of provision of single-use injection equipment. The effectiveness of interventions to reduce injection frequency was highly variable (1–53%) due to the variability in approaches and study designs. In our model, we used the estimate of effectiveness reported for interactional group discussions (30%) – a well-designed, well-evaluated intervention that has been used in developing countries (Prawitasari Hadiyono et al. 1996). Interactional group discussions consist of moderated patient–prescriber discussions on the topic of injection use, during which the prescribers are confronted with the actual absence of preference for injections among patients.

Our disease model was based on the number of contaminated injections – a product of the number of injections received and the proportion of these given with reused equipment. Thus, we assumed that the effectiveness of the combined interventions was a multiplication of the effect of the two. In the absence of evidence suggesting the contrary, we also assumed that intervention effectiveness did not differ with respect to the underlying magnitude of the burden under the 'do nothing' scenario.

Cost of interventions

First, we identified the activities required for each intervention at the national and subnational level for an implementation period of ten years. Each of these activities was assigned to the intervention to reduce injection use or to the intervention to reduce unsafe practices, or both (in the case of the latter, activities necessary in the two interventions were counted only once). We then estimated the quantity of fulltime-equivalent staff members and the material resources required to conduct these activities. Third, we estimated the needs of single-use syringe and needle sets on the basis of the number of injections administered and the proportion already given using sterile injection equipment. Fourth, the resources required for safe sharps waste collection and management were taken into account as part of the intervention. The needs quantified for ten years were then averaged to obtain a yearly estimate that we used to cost the hypothetical intervention in the year 2000.

We estimated the average yearly programme cost for human resources and associated materials for the year 2000 by costing studies conducted in each subregion as part of the WHOCHOICE project. The cost of injection equipment was calculated on the basis of international retail prices and the cost of distribution. First, we estimated international retail market prices among main international wholesalers. Second, we estimated international distribution costs on a standardized mark-up. Third, we estimated the cost of domestic distribution on the basis of a model that calculated the distances between the theoretical centre of a country with the highest population densities and a periphery with the lowest population density. The cost of personnel, capital, and fuel was estimated from a database to which fuel efficiency and maintenance cost was added. Finally, we used costing studies conducted by WHO to estimate the costs per syringe and needle set of sharps waste collection and disposal through incineration. All costs were expressed in international dollars (I$) for the year 2000. An international dollar has the same purchasing power as the US dollar has in the United States, and is derived via the application of purchasing power parity exchange rates. We assumed 100% coverage of all situations where injections were given in the formal public sector (e.g. hospitals, clinics).

Uncertainty analysis

We first tested the upper and lower values of the attributable fraction of the comparative risk assessment. Second, we assumed that the effectiveness of interventions was only 7% for reducing injection use (the lowest effectiveness reported for an intervention targeting patients and providers) and 50% for reducing unsafe use of injections. Third, we ran the analysis using an upper value of the number of syringes and needle sets required. Fourth, we ran an analysis that did not take into account the additional cost of safe sharps waste collection and management. Finally, total estimated costs and effects were simulated in a stochastic uncertainty analysis of the probability that interventions represent a cost-effective use of resources given a specified budget constraint.

Results

Effectiveness of interventions

The number of injections per person per year was estimated to range from 1.7 in AMR B to 11.3 in EUR C, of which a proportion ranging from 1.2% in EUR B and 75% in SEAR D was administered with injection equipment reused in the absence of sterilization (Table 17.3). Overall, contaminated injections caused 21 million HBV infections, two million HCV infections and 260 000 HIV infections. These infections led to 49 000, 24 000, and 210 000 deaths, respectively, between the years 2000 and 2030, for a total of 9 177 679 discounted and age-weighted DALYs (non-discounted, unadjusted DALYs, 48 541 032). HIV infections accounted for the highest proportion of DALYs (63%), whereas HBV and HCV infections accounted for 34% and 4% of the total, respectively. Most of this burden was caused by early death rather than by disability.

The assumed effectiveness of interactional group discussion translated directly into projected burden of disease reduction as the incidence of injection-associated infections in the present disease model was proportional to the annual number of injections per person and the proportion of injections given with reused equipment. Implementation of interventions to reduce injection use would lead to a reduction of 2 753 304 DALYs. The effectiveness of provision of single use injection equipment was assumed to be 95% on the unsafe use of injections. Implementation of interventions to reduce the unsafe use of injections would lead to a reduction of 8 718 795 DALYs. When combined, the two interventions would lead to a reduction of 8 856 461 DALYs.

Costs of interventions

The expected annual cost of the intervention to reduce injection use ranged from I$ 0.009 per capita in AMR D to I$ 0.024 in WPR B. The cost per capita of the intervention to reduce the unsafe use of injections ranged from I$ 0.01 in AMR D to I$ 0.44 in SEAR D. A high proportion of these costs (83–99% in all subregions other than AMR B and EUR B) consisted of injection equipment, including international retail price, international transport, and waste management. Overall, the international retail price accounted for 40% of the total injection equipment costs. The estimated yearly cost per capita of combined interventions ranged from I$ 0.03 in AMR D to I$ 0.45 in SEAR D.

Cost-effectiveness of interventions

The average cost-effectiveness ratio (CER; total costs divided by total effects) for interventions to reduce injection use was I$ 7 to I$ 5124 per DALY averted according to the region (Table 17.4). The average CER for interventions to reduce unsafe use of injections, including waste management, was I$ 12 to I$ 1107 per DALY averted according to the region. The average CER for combined interventions for the safe and appropriate use of injections, including waste management, was I$ 14 to I$ 2293 per DALY averted according to the region. Incremental analysis suggested that in the six subregions in which the proportion of reuse of injection equipment exceeds 15%, the intervention to reduce injection use represents the single most cost-effective strategy. In the four other subregions, the reduction of unsafe use was the most efficient strategy. However, in all regions, the average CER of the combined intervention strategy remained under the threshold of one year of average per capita income.

Uncertainty analysis

Five scenarios were assessed in the sensitivity analysis (Table 17.5). Higher attributable fraction reduced the average cost per DALY averted by 19–86% compared with the base case, but removing the costs of sharps waste management had little additional influence on baseline results (scenarios 1 and 2, with the latter representing the best case). Attribution of a lower fraction of injection-related infections raised the average cost per DALY averted (scenario 3). Using the minimum estimates for intervention effectiveness in addition to the lower attributable fractions increased CER ratios further, particularly for the intervention to reduce injection use (scenario 4). Finally, a scenario incorporating the lower attributable fraction, minimum effectiveness, and a doubled number of syringe and needle sets (scenario 5) resulted in a four- to ten-fold increase in the average cost per DALY averted, compared with initial baseline estimates. However, even in this worst-case scenario, the average cost-effectiveness ratio of all interventions remained below the threshold of average annual income per capita. Inclusion of best- and worst-case total costs and effects in the stochastic uncertainty analysis showed that at very low levels of resource availability, reduction of injection use represents the most cost-effective strategy in most subregions (a small health gain, but achieved at a low cost). At higher levels of resource availability, a combination approach would be the most efficient choice (considerably greater health gains at an increased but still cost-effective level of investment).

Table 17.4 Costs and cost-effectiveness of policies for the safe and appropriate use of injections

	African region		Region of the Americas		Eastern Mediterranean	European region		South-East Asia region		Western Pacific
	AFR D	AFR E	AMR B	AMR D	EMR D	EUR B	EUR C	SEAR B	SEAR D	WPR B
Total population (million)	294	346	431	71	343	218	243	294	1 242	1 533
Gross domestic product per capita	1 381	1 576	7 833	3 837	2 393	7 294	6 916	2 545	1 449	4 186
Syringes/needles costs¹ (I$ million)	19.18	18.21	1.12	2.08	148.49	0.77	11.42	25.54	454.50	144 59
Programme costs²										
Reduction of injection use	2.74	3.31	10.52	1.08	3.88	5.35	5.30	3.57	10.60	25.58
Reduction of unsafe use	1.60	19.60	3.19	0.43	1.54	2.88	1.69	1.22	4.40	8.45
Combination	3.55	21.92	11.02	1.21	4.23	6.92	5.55	3.76	11.81	27.16
Average CER (I$ per DALY averted)										
Reduction of injection use	16	7	3 862	132	23	5 124	273	42	7	66
Reduction of unsafe use	39	12	499	97	282	1 107	213	100	102	125
Combined interventions	42	14	1 385	125	283	2 293	272	108	102	138
Incremental CER (I$ per DALY averted)										
Reduction of injection use	16	7	–	–	23	–	–	42	7	66
Reduction of unsafe use	50	15	499	97	–	1 107	213	127	–	152
Combined interventions	234	93	57 579	1 882	400	77 666	3 977	603	145	969

1 Includes international retail price, international transport and waste management
2 Includes personnel, transport, equipment, and supplies (excluding syringes and needles)

Source: Dziekan et al. (2003)

Table 17.5 Sensitivity analysis

Sensitivity scenario	African region		Region of the Americas		Eastern Mediterranean	European region		South-East Asia region		Western Pacific
	AFR D	AFR E	AMR B	AMR D	EMR D	EUR B	EUR C	SEAR B	SEAR D	WPR B
Higher attributable fraction[1]										
Reduction of injection use	13	5	523	44	17	1 394	140	33	6	28
Reduction of unsafe use	32	10	68	33	210	301	109	79	78	53
Combination	34	11	187	42	210	624	139	85	78	59
Higher attributable fraction, no sharps waste management										
Reduction of injection use	13	5	523	44	17	1 394	140	33	6	28
Reduction of unsafe use	20	6	61	22	127	276	71	49	47	33
Combination	23	7	181	31	129	599	102	55	48	39
Lower attributable fraction										
Reduction of injection use	22	9	NA[2]	NA	45	NA	970	57	11	NA
Reduction of unsafe use	52	16	NA	NA	544	NA	758	136	156	NA
Combination	56	18	NA	NA	546	NA	967	146	156	NA
Lower attributable fraction, minimum effectiveness										
Reduction of injection use	93	37	NA	NA	191	NA	4 159	245	49	NA
Reduction of unsafe use	99	31	NA	NA	1 035	NA	1 441	258	296	NA
Combination	106	34	NA	NA	1 038	NA	1 838	278	296	NA
Lower attributable fraction, minimum effect, double injection sets										
Reduction of injection use	93	37	NA	NA	191	NA	4 159	245	49	NA
Reduction of unsafe use	190	60	NA	NA	2 058	NA	2 696	504	589	NA
Combination	196	62	NA	NA	2 046	NA	3 074	520	585	NA

1 Attributable fraction refers to the fraction of new Hepatitis B, Hepatitis C and HIV infections attributable to contaminated injections
2 NA not applicable lower attributable fraction equals zero

Source: Dziekan et al. (2003)

Limitations

First, the model did not take into account any longer-term dynamic effects that reducing transmission of infection would have on the prevalence of infections with bloodborne pathogens. This could be a problem in the case of HCV infection because contaminated injections account for a high proportion of new infections. This limitation could also lead to an underestimation of the effect size, hence these interventions might be described as being less cost-effective than they really are. Second, the specific issues associated with working in the private sector were not addressed. The provision of sufficient quantities of single-use injection equipment and interactional group discussion might not be sufficient where the informal private sector accounts for a high proportion of healthcare services delivery. In such settings, demonstration projects should identify effective strategies, some of which might include the use of AD syringes in curative services or addressing financial incentives to overprescribing injections, or both.

 Feedback

> You should have concluded that this study was fairly well conducted and reported. Most items, where relevant, were addressed. However, the viewpoint of the study was not clearly stated and justified (it appears to have been undertaken from the perspective of a health care provider). Perhaps the least satisfactory part of the study relates to the estimates of the effectiveness of the interventions. More justification might have been provided for the assumptions made.

How good does a study have to be to be useful?

Few studies will meet all the criteria with respect to conduct and reporting. Indeed this is as it should be since the marginal cost of the additional effort to produce perfection is likely to be greater than the marginal benefit from further improvements to an already good study. Analytical resources are scarce and any incremental effort to improve one study has an opportunity cost in benefits foregone from other evaluations.

As a consequence, despite these well-established and widely used checklists, the critical appraisal of economic evaluations will depend on the context in which the evaluation is taking place. While different assessors should be able to reach agreement on how a particular study performs with respect to each item, they might very well disagree with respect to a global assessment of the quality and relevance of a particular study.

On occasion a decision-maker might simply be concerned with whether or not a particular study is of sufficient quality that it can directly inform a decision. However, no single study adequately addresses a decision-maker's concerns – a synthesis of several studies is needed. The issue is then how to combine information from these different sources and when to give greater weight to particular studies.

This raises the general question as to what quality is required for a study to be useful and how to judge the quality of one study *vis-à-vis* that of another. How important are the different aspects of quality? To what extent can higher quality with respect to one aspect compensate for lower quality with respect to another? There are no simple answers to these questions, depending, as they do, on the preferences of the users of evaluations.

Summary

You have learnt about the key attributes of an economic evaluation that need to be considered when judging its quality. This has become more detailed and sophisticated over time. There are three main aspects to consider: study design; data collection; and the analysis and interpretation of the results.

References

Drummond MF and Jefferson TO (1996) Guidelines for authors and peer reviewers of economic submissions to the BMJ. *British Medical Journal* 313:275.

Drummond MF, Stoddart GL and Torrance GW (1987) *Methods for the economic evaluation of health care programmes.* Oxford: Oxford University Press.

Dzeikan G, Chisolm D, Johns B, Rovira J and Hutin YJF (2003) The cost-effectiveness of policies for the safe and appropriate use of injection in healthcare settings. *Bulletin of the World Health Organization* 81(4):277–285, www.who.int/bulletin/en.

Prawitasari Hadiyono JE, Suryawati S, Danu SS, Sunartono and Santoso B (1996) Interactional group discussion: results of a controlled trial using a behavioural intervention to reduce the use of injections in public health facilities. *Social Science & Medicine* 42:1177–83.

Further reading

The following website provides a useful database of economic evaluations and for many of them provides a critical appraisal: www.york.ac.uk/inst/crd/crddatabases.htm.

18 Transferring cost-effectiveness data across space and time

Overview

Increasing demand from decision-makers for cost-effectiveness analyses, coupled with limited research resources and a paucity of evidence is creating pressure to transfer data across settings. The desire to extrapolate results occurs both within and between countries. However, as you will learn in this chapter, transferring economic data is often problematic. You will learn how to transfer results between different geographical places, from randomized trials to routine settings and over time, as well as some of the problems encountered.

Learning objectives

By the end of this chapter, you will be able to:

- **understand the importance of transferring costs, effects and cost-effectiveness results from one setting to another**
- **critically appraise methods for transferring cost and effectiveness data from one setting to another**
- **use simple techniques to transfer cost data from one setting to another**
- **understand the concept of purchasing power parities and other relative price indices for comparing the results of economic evaluations**

Key terms

External validity (generalisability) The extent to which the results of a study can be generalised to the population from which the sample was drawn.

Internal validity (of a model) Accuracy and consistency of underpinning mathematical calculations with the specifications of the model.

International dollar The same purchasing power as the US dollar in the United States.

Non-traded goods Services and commodities which cannot be traded on the international market. Therefore the cost or price is likely to vary across regions. Examples include utilities, buildings, domestic transport and some types of labour.

Study protocol A plan with complete details on the conduct of a study including tests, medications and procedures as well as study design.

Traded goods Commodities that are available on the international market. In theory, all countries can purchase them at an international market price.

Transferability The extent to which the results of a study as it applies to a particular patient group or setting hold true for another population or context.

Introduction

The growing need for economic evidence to inform resource allocation decisions has led many to question the extent to which the results and conclusions of a study carried out in one setting can be extrapolated to other contexts. In other words, how transferable are the results?

In this chapter you will explore how costs, effects and cost-effectiveness ratios can be most appropriately transferred across settings. It is useful at this stage to think of transferring results in two ways: transferring the entire result of economic evaluations and transferring the individual parts of the cost-effectiveness ratio. You will learn about both of these situations.

You will start by considering some of the key issues in transferring the results of economic evaluations before examining basic methods for transferring cost-effectiveness ratios over space and time. You will then explore methods for transferring unit costs between geographical settings and issues concerning transferring effects. Finally, you will explore how studies could be better designed to improve the transferability of results.

Challenges for transferability

You know that the results of economic evaluations depend on a wide range of highly localized factors. In addition there are considerable international differences in the practice of health care itself, which are often even greater than those differences within a single system. For example, doctors trained in different health systems are likely to prescribe different drugs and procedures for the same condition and a hospital stay for treatment of a given condition cannot be assumed to involve the same inputs.

Health systems are characterized by different levels and types of resources, which implies that care regimens offered within one health system may not be offered within another. Different prices apply and this implies not only that costs differ for an identical package of care but also that the most economically efficient way of delivering care varies. For example, where labour is cheap, efficient production techniques will be more labour intensive.

Health systems are also organized differently. For example, specialist doctors have traditionally taken responsibility for much primary care in the US and France whereas generalist doctors play the same role in Canada and the UK, and other health care workers with more limited training may have much of this responsibility in low-income countries.

Population and demographic characteristics also affect results. A programme to identify and screen for cataracts is more costly to deliver in a remote village in

Nepal than it is in the densely populated capital of Kathmandu. It is also clear that effectiveness will depend on the underlying disease conditions.

All of the above suggests that, at best, you need to consider carefully the results of economic evaluations undertaken in different settings to your own. At worst, it means that using the international literature for evidence of cost-effectiveness relevant to choices to be made in a specific country may be seriously misleading.

Activity 18.1

Give examples of how the following can limit the transferability of economic results between settings:

1 Basic demography and epidemiology of disease.
2 Availability of health care resources (e.g. capital, labour).
3 Incentives to health care professionals.
4 Clinical practice (including skills).

Feedback

1 Vaccination and screening programmes are likely to be more cost-effective in populations where the incidence of the particular disease under study is high. Different age structures between countries are likely to lead to different levels of incidence in various countries and therefore to different levels of disease burden.

2 In some countries with national health care systems, such as Italy or UK, access to services is controlled by rationing in the form of waiting lists for hospital admission, whereas in private insurance systems rationing is by ability to pay.

3 Doctors who are paid a fee for service are more likely to generate extra demand for their services, whereas those paid by salary may be more likely to look for ways to reduce the demand for health services. Both behaviours will affect the care provided and, therefore, total costs.

4 Clinicians can influence the effectiveness and cost-effectiveness of interventions. In certain types of surgical treatment the effect of the clinician is an integral part of the treatment. With such interventions, variation in the skill and experience of the clinician can have a substantial effect on the process of care and the outcomes.

Methods for transferring costs and effects

You saw in Chapter 16 that the most common format for presenting the outcome of economic evaluations is to show the ICERs of the status quo (do nothing option) through to better but more expensive options. The ICER is the extra cost of the additional service divided by the extra outcome of effectiveness.

Figure 18.1 shows how the ICER is built upon a comparison of the total costs and total effects of two interventions. Total costs are a function of price (p) and quantity (q) of inputs. Total effects are a function of value (v) placed on the change in health

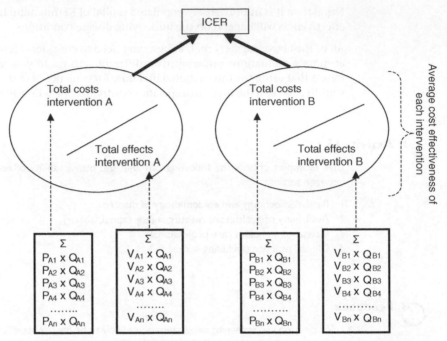

Figure 18.1 Components in an economic evaluation for transferring across time or space

benefit (for CUAs) and the 'quantity' (q) of the effect (it could be quantity or quality of life). Before dealing with variation in either the costs or the effects, the first concern of analysts is to ensure that the overall results are presented in a way that is comparable. Two initial tasks are therefore to express costs in a common currency and for the same period, which affect P_{An} and P_{Bn} in Figure 18.1.

Expressing results in a common currency

The usual practice is to convert costs into a common currency (such as the US dollar) using official exchange rates. However, these rates do not necessarily reflect the relative purchasing power of different currencies as one unit of a common currency may buy different quantities of the same item in different countries. Purchasing power parities (PPPs) are rates of currency conversion that equalize purchasing power of different currencies. That is, they attempt to eliminate the differences in price levels for the same goods between countries. Often the results from multinational comparisons are presented in international dollars using PPP exchange rates. An international dollar has the same purchasing power as the US dollar has in the United States. Costs in local currency units are converted to international dollars using PPP exchange rates. Whilst international dollars are the most frequently encountered currency, it would be possible to use any other currency as the base.

Some economists argue that wherever possible PPPs should be specific to health care goods and services to obtain an accurate reflection of the relative cost of health care interventions. One of the reasons is because labour tends to have higher inflationary pressures than goods and labour tends to be a high proportion of health services.

To convert international dollars to local currency, simply multiply the international dollar figure by the PPP exchange conversion factor. To convert local currency units to international dollars, divide the local currency unit by the PPP conversion factor.

Transferring costs over time

As price levels increase over time (or in rarer instances, decrease) there is a need to adjust cost information when comparing data from different years. If the unit price of a drug was $1.00 last year and $1.05 this year, this reflects an increase in the real resources used if the inflation was less than the percent change in price, i.e. less than 5%. If inflation were only 4%, the drug price has increased by 1% more than inflation. On the other hand, if inflation were 11%, there would have been a 6% reduction in the price of drugs relative to inflation over time. Thus in order to compare across years (or to convert the value of resources to one given year), costs need to be expressed in the same values. This conversion is done using measures of domestic inflation such as consumer price indices or gross domestic product (GDP) deflators.

The following are two commonly used indices for converting prices to the same year:

- *consumer price index (CPI)* reflects the change in the cost to the average consumer of purchasing a fixed basket of goods and services;
- *The GDP* price deflator is a price index that measures the change in the price level of GDP relative to real output. In other words, it measures the average annual rate of price change in the economy as a whole.

To convert expenditure in year Y to the prices of the chosen base year X, multiply the expenditure in year Y by, for example, the consumer price index for the base year X and divide by the consumer price index for year Y.

In multinational studies, you may want to compare costs over time across several different countries. Because inflation rates are likely to differ, especially in relation to the US (if an international dollar is used for comparison), it is better to work in local currencies first and then convert to US dollars or international dollars at the end.

Transferring unit costs

While the methods described above are adequate for expressing total costs in a common currency and for transferring costs over time, they still assume that the *type* and *quantity* of inputs going into the intervention are the same across settings. However, for reasons outlined earlier this is unlikely to be the case. For example, differences in labour costs may affect the relative cost-effectiveness of inpatient and day surgery. Therefore, analysts have found ways for allowing for differences in the *unit costs* of interventions between different settings where you might expect relative prices and inputs to differ. These approaches change the value of individual units costs (e.g. $P_{A1} \times Q_{A1}$ in Figure 18.1) or groups of unit costs (e.g. $P_{B1} \times Q_{B1} + P_{B2} \times Q_{B2}$ in Figure 18.1).

Perhaps the most important contribution to this area at the international level has been the development of standardized costs for the World Health Organization in the form of a database called WHO-CHOICE available on the internet at www.whochoice.who.org. In response to the lack of reliable estimates on the unit costs of health care in many countries, the World Health Organization used cost data collected from many countries to predict unit costs in countries for which data are not available. These costs were then aggregated to form average standard costs for whole regions such as sub-Saharan Africa and South Asia. Other global initiatives using standardized costs include the Commission for Macro-economics and Health (www.cmhealth.org/) and, more recently, the Disease Control Priorities Project (www.fic.nih.gov/dcpp/). At the national level there have been various developments. For example, the UK National Health Service has developed a set of national reference costs that provide average cost of treatments, procedures and care across a range of hospitals. There also exists a national dataset on the unit costs of delivering personal and social care services.

The various methods employed in the literature for transferring unit costs can be broadly divided into regression-based approaches and standardization approaches. Regression-based methods include models that attempt to explain how costs per unit of activity vary in relation to a variety of variables such as hospital size, service mix, input prices and average length of stay. The results can then be used to predict unit costs for settings where data on unit cost is missing. This was the approach adopted by WHO-CHOICE (Adam *et al.* 2003). A disadvantage of this approach, however, is that it relies on a great deal of data. In addition, very few studies have attempted to explain differences in unit costs at the country level. A different approach, standardized indices, is potentially less data 'hungry'. It develops a relative cost index. One example of this approach is provided by Schulman *et al.* (1998) who developed an index table using a market-based approach reflecting the relative costs. Often, unit costs may not be available for some sites in a study. In this situation a standardized costing methodology can be developed from countries where there are data. This is a more transparent method for adjusting cost data from one setting to another.

Schulman *et al.* developed a standardized costing methodology in seven countries and applied it to the costing of treatments for subarachnoid haemorrhage. Where unit cost estimates were not available they developed an index table based on a market-basket approach reflecting the relative costs of a basket of resources for six services for which unit cost data were available for all countries (see Table 18.1). To estimate the cost of a given procedure for a given country the relative weight is simply applied to the unit cost of the source country. The table is read from the left to right, so moving data from Sweden to France would be 0.68 and not 1.47.

Table 18.1 Relative medical cost indices of the study countries

Index	Germany	Italy	France	Sweden	UK	Australia
Germany	1.00	1.35	1.35	2.64	2.41	2.03
Italy	0.74	1.00	1.33	1.96	1.79	1.51
France	0.56	0.75	1.00	1.47	1.34	1.13
Sweden	0.38	0.51	0.68	1.00	0.77	0.73
UK	0.42	0.56	0.75	1.10	1.00	0.84
Australia	0.49	0.66	0.88	1.30	1.19	1.00

Source: Schulman *et al.* (1998)

 Activity 18.2

You are provided with unit cost information from a study conducted in Italy. The data are all for the year 2004 and you are told that the Italian CPI for 2004 and 2005 is 121 and 123 respectively. The costs in US$ are as follows: craniofacial procedures (471); dialysis (206); gastroscopy (245); one-day in intensive care (601); and one-day in intermediate care (304).

1 Convert the above unit costs into prices for 2005.
2 Using the information in Table 18.1, estimate the equivalent unit costs for Germany for 2004 and 2005.
3 Describe some of the possible reasons for the variation in the estimated unit costs.

 Feedback

1 Compare your results with these: craniofacial procedures (479); dialysis (209); gastroscopy (249); one-day in intensive care (611); and one-day in intermediate care (309). An example calculation for dialysis is $(206 \times 123)/121 = 209$.

2 The appropriate index to use for Germany is 0.74. An example calculation for craniofacial procedures in 2004 is $0.74 \times 471 = 349$. Transferring data to Germany for 2005 requires using the answers to question 1.

3 Possible reasons for the variation include differences in the determinants of cost such as the technology involved in production, the rate of substitution between labour and capital and the types and cost of resource inputs, which are likely to vary. Variation in the purchasing power of different currencies is another reason because the costs are expressed in US dollars and not PPP exchange dollars.

Dealing with traded and non-traded inputs

Ideally, studies done in one country should show the quantities and prices of inputs in their setting. Analysts in other settings can simply adjust the quantities and prices as needed. However, it is more often the case that analysts do not have the price and cost information. The next best method is to make a distinction between traded and non-traded goods. This is another approach that impacts on the Ps in Figure 18.1.

Traded goods are commodities that are available on the international market and, in theory, all countries can purchase them at an international market price. The international price can therefore be considered to reflect the opportunity cost of purchasing traded goods to a country without price distortions, adjusted to include carriage, insurance and freight for imported goods. It is worth noting that while an international price may exist, there are still substantial differences in the prices actually paid for traded goods, particularly drugs, even after accounting for taxes. This is due to, for example, economies of scale in production or special price agreements (e.g. for HIV/AIDS drugs).

In contrast to traded goods, the price of non-traded and mixed goods like labour, utilities, buildings and domestic transport are likely to vary across countries. In many instances the distinction between traded and non-traded is not so straight-forward and most inputs are made up of a traded and non-traded component.

The most common situation is where input prices are not available and the traded and non-traded components are unknown. An example of this situation may be the unit cost per inpatient day or the unit cost of a particular procedure. In these cases some kind of relative price index as described above can be used to translate unit costs from one setting to another.

 Activity 18.3

List which of the following components of a laboratory test you think are traded between countries and which are not traded between countries. Explain your answers:

- equipment
- labour
- drugs and supplies
- office space

 Feedback

Equipment, drugs and supplies are classified as traded goods as they can be traded on the international market and, in theory, an international price should exist. Labour and office space on the other hand cannot be (easily) traded internationally. However, it is possible to argue that for some highly specialist labour (such as doctors) there may exist an international price and workers can move from country to country.

Transferring effects

Randomized trials are the most reliable way to determine the effect of interventions. They tend to have concentrated on producing unbiased estimates of effect in the trial sample, with little regard to how the results might be relevant to other population groups. This might be because biological responses are assumed to be universal, i.e. the clinical effect of a patient taking a given drug is expected to be similar in the UK and Australia. However, this view does not account for the possibility that clinical and health end-points may not be independent of the health care setting.

Rothwell (2005) worked through a whole range of reasons why clinical results may not transfer across settings, many of which are covered earlier in this chapter. However, health care provided in a trial may differ from routine practice. For example, the relevance and appropriateness of the control arm is of key importance. If the control arm is different to routine practice, then any estimation of effect size based on the difference between intervention and control cannot necessarily be deemed to transfer to current practice (indeed, even discussion of how comparable the control arm data is within international trials is often avoided). Trials may also become out of date as new therapeutic procedures are developed and are therefore not transferable over time. Much care also needs to be given to check how readily the characteristics of patients apply to other settings. This would include comparisons of severity of disease, co-morbidity, age, sex and racial group.

Data on effect sizes from randomized trials can be presented in a number of ways – for example, absolute or relative risk (benefit) reductions. An absolute risk is the risk of developing a disease (or event) over a specific time period and for a specific population. Relative risk is used to compare the risk in two different groups of people in a specified time period. For example, the groups could be 'smokers' and 'non-smokers' or control/trial arms in a randomized trial. Quantifying baseline health effects of existing treatments separately from the relative effects of new health interventions is a useful way of estimating absolute health effects. It is also useful for adjusting absolute effects to other population groups (NICE 2004) and is the process by which Q_{An} and Q_{Bn} in Figure 18.1 might be transferred.

There have been several approaches to considering how widely applicable the results of randomized trials are. First, there has been some attempt to undertake 'pragmatic' trials that have as few exclusion criteria as possible and try to follow routine care as much as possible. Second, systematic reviews are conducted to ensure that as much evidence as possible is collated and considered as a whole (or excluding papers rated below some quality threshold).

The Cochrane Collaboration is a non-profit organization that produces and disseminates systematic reviews of health care interventions using evidence from over 90 countries. Its name commemorates the work and collaborative principles of the British epidemiologist Archie Cochrane. It has a particular (but not exclusive) focus on synthesizing evidence from randomized trials and, if studies are shown to be relatively similar (e.g. in terms of interventions, populations and patient characteristics), a statistical meta-analysis can be undertaken to calculate a summary estimate of the size of effect of treatment. The selection of studies is key to ensuring results are not biased and researchers are encouraged to contact the Cochrane Collaboration in developing study protocols. In the space of ten years, 2000 systematic reviews have been completed and their results have already had an impact on clinical practice guidelines and in some instances on clinical practice. Donaldson *et al.* (2002) have written about how the evidence produced in such systematic reviews can be used in economic evaluations as well as setting a research agenda.

There are also good reasons to believe that not only might the quantity of health effect vary by setting but also the *value* placed on absolute and relative benefits by patients. As you saw in Chapter 9, the EuroQol group has provided different valuations for the same health states in around 15 countries. This is the process by which V_{An} and V_{Bn} in Figure 18.1 might be transferred and such differences might change the interpretation of RCTs in different contexts (Rothwell 2005).

Designing studies in the future

The aim of economic evaluation is to support decision-making and you have seen some of the challenges of transferring the results of economic evaluations to other settings. Perhaps a better approach would be to design and undertake economic evaluations to take account of these transferability issues. Sculpher *et al.* (2004) conclude that there are at least three opportunities to increase the transferability of economic studies undertaken in the future.

First, it should be possible to anticipate the need for generalizability of findings at the design stage. An important recommendation here is to collect resource use data (e.g. hospital days, intensive care unit days etc.) separately from the unit costs or prices of those resources. This allows decision-makers considering a study undertaken in another location to assess whether the practice patterns seen in the study apply to their own setting. Furthermore, they can apply their own prices to the unit of resource use.

A second opportunity for enhancing the transferability of results is in the analysis of results to produce findings relevant to a range of settings. A number of statistical and econometric approaches examining the nature of variability in costs, effects and cost-effectiveness by location have been explored in the literature and this is the subject of ongoing research.

The 'generalized cost-effectiveness analysis' (Tan-Torres *et al.* 2003) is a different approach to enhancing the transferability of economic evaluations by using cost-effectiveness analysis to provide generic information on the relative costs and effects of different health interventions in the absence of local decision constraints. It involves the evaluation of the costs and benefits of a set of related interventions with respect to a 'do nothing' option. According to proponents of the approach, this provides a complete set of information for identifying the health maximizing combination of interventions for any given budget. The results are presented in a single league table. For each set of mutually exclusive interventions, the intervention with the lowest cost-effectiveness ratio when compared with the 'do nothing' option would appear the most attractive. The second intervention from the set that appears in the league table represents the incremental cost-effectiveness ratio with respect to the first. By analysing the costs and effects of mutually exclusive interventions with respect to a 'do nothing' approach, the results are considered to be more transferable from one population to another. Critics of the approach argue that considering a 'do nothing' option is problematic given that it depends on the local health system in place, demographic and epidemiological circumstances and the development of models documenting the natural history of disease in the absence of interventions.

The third opportunity raised by Schulpher *et al.* (2004) is in the reporting of results, where analysts ideally should try to reflect the needs of decision-makers in different geographical locations. They argue that even if it has not been possible to address fully all the issues of transferability at the design or analysis stage, economic evaluations should accommodate the needs of study users in the reporting of results. For example, the study site should be clearly described and the perspective adopted should be clear to the reader to help the users of studies decide whether a given study is relevant to their own setting.

 Activity 18.4

Go back and review the paper by Dziekan *et al.* that you read in Chapter 17. Consider whether the results would be relevant to your setting. What adjustments do you think are necessary? The following questions are useful issues to consider (Heyland *et al.* 1996).

1 Are the patients described in the analysis similar to those patients in your setting?
2 Is the intervention under study generalizable to your setting?
3 Are the costing methods applicable to the health care system in which you work?
4 Is the unit price for drugs, physician fees, laboratory tests etc. the same?
5 Is the mix of resources consumed the same?
6 Is the volume of patients, and therefore the average cost per patient, similar across systems?
7 Can you convert exchange rates across systems appropriately?
8 Are the outcomes measured appropriately for your setting?
9 Was a method to measure the outcomes compatible with the current methods utilized in your setting?
10 If a preference-based measure was used, is there evidence that the preferences of your patients are the same as those preferences used in the analysis?
11 Is the discount rate applicable to your setting?

Feedback

1 The results of the evaluation are provided for all 14 World Health Organization regions (based on burden of disease) so it is likely that a region, which has a similar disease profile to your own, can be identified.

2 The interventions under study are well described, so you should be able to make a judgement as to whether it is generalizable to your setting.

3–6 This is a 'generalized' cost-effectiveness analysis, which assumes a baseline do nothing approach. You will need to consider whether your health system is typical of those characterized by the selected sub-region. The intervention costs themselves are based on World Health Organization costing studies undertaken in each sub-region. You may need to review local data and/or literature to determine how typical they are of costs in your setting and whether the mix of resources consumed is the same. The average cost per patient is based on regional population data and therefore the results should be comparable across systems.

7 PPPs were used to convert costs, which helps comparison of costs between countries.

8–10 Outcomes were measured using DALYs, which facilitates comparisons across settings and disease areas. To make adjustments to effectiveness you would need to re-estimate the model using different baseline estimates of needle use and the effectiveness of the programmes. It may also be appropriate to use a different underlying mortality rate as most benefits were related to life years gained. If preference values differ it is unlikely to have a significant impact as most benefits were in terms of mortality gain, but preference value changes are most likely to have an impact on the European regions.

11 The discount rate used was 3% which may be different to rates in some countries, particularly those that have faced any recent financial shocks. Overall, the further away a country is from any average regional estimate, particularly for influential variables, the more likely results will be affected.

Summary

You have learnt how estimates of costs, effectiveness and cost-effectiveness ratios can be most appropriately transferred across settings. You saw the need to express results in a common currency and to consider the challenge of transferring results over time. You will now go on to look at how economic evaluations are used in practice and policy.

References

Adam T, Evans DB and Murray CJL (2003) Econometric estimation of country-specific hospital costs. *Cost Effectiveness and Resource Allocation* 1:3, www.resource-allocation.com/content/1/1/3/.

Donaldson D, Mugford M and Vale L (2002) *Evidence-based health economics: from effectiveness to efficiency in systematic review*. London: BMJ Books.

Heyland DK, Kernerman P, Gafni A and Cook DJ (1996) Economic evaluations in the critical care literature: do they help is improve the efficiency of our unit? *Critical Care Medicine* 24:1591–8.

NICE (2004) *Guide to the methods of technology appraisal*. London: NICE, www.nice.org.uk.

Rothwell PM (2005) External validity of randomized controlled trials: 'To whom do the results of this trial apply?' *The Lancet*, 365:82–93.

Schulman K, Burke UJ, Drummond M, Davies L, Carlsson P, Gruger J, Harris A, Lucioni A, Gisbert R, Llana T, Tom E, Bloom B, Willke R and Glick H (1998) Resource costing for multinational neurological clinical trials: methods and results. *Health Economics* 7:629–38.

Sculpher ML, Pang FS, Manca FA, Drummond MF, Golder S, Urdhal H, Davies LM and Eastwood A (2004) Generalisability in economic evaluation studies in health care: a review and case studies. *Health Technology Assessment* 18(49), www.ncchta.org/fullmono/mon849.pdf.

Tan-Torres Edejer T, Baltussen R, Adam T, Hutubessy R, Acharya A, Evans DB and Murray CJL (2003) *Making choices in health: WHO guide to cost-effectiveness analysis*. Geneva: WHO. See also details on WHO-CHOICE project on www.who.int/evidence/cea.

Further reading

Cochrane reviews are based on the best available information about health care interventions. They explore the evidence for and against the effectiveness and appropriateness of treatments (medications, surgery, education etc.) in specific circumstances. The library for reproductive health is free to developing countries. See www.cochrane.org/index0.htm.

Curtis L and Netten A (2004) *Unit costs of health and social care*, www.pssru.ac.uk/uc/uc2004.htm.

Kumaranayake L (2000) The real and the nominal? Making inflationary adjustments to cost and other economic data. *Health Policy & Planning* 15(2):230–4, http://heapol.oupjournals.org/search.dtl.

Mulligan J, Fox-Rushby J, Adam T, Johns B and Mills A (2003) *Unit costs of health care inputs in low and middle income regions*. DCPP Working Paper No. 9, September, www.fic.nih.gov/dcpp/wps/wp9.pdf.

NHS reference costs and national tariff can be found in a series of documents on the following website: www.dh.gov.uk/PublicationsAndStatistics/Publications/PublicationsPolicyAndGuidance/PublicationsPolicyAndGuidanceArticle/fs/en?CONTENT_ID=4070195&chk=UzhHA3.

WHO CHOICE: http://www3.who.int/whosis/menu.cfm?path=evidence,cea&language=english.

World Bank: www.worldbank.org/.

Use of economic evaluation in practice and policy

Overview

In this chapter you will learn about the use of economic evaluation at international, national and sub-national levels in setting health care policy and influencing practice. It identifies some of the shortcomings of published economic evaluations and explores barriers to using economic evaluation more widely. Finally, the chapter reflects on some ways of improving the use and usefulness of economic evaluations in the future.

Learning objectives

After working through this chapter, you will be able to:

- **distinguish between the methodology and practice of economic evaluations**
- **understand the uses of economic evidence in policy**
- **describe with examples how economic evaluations are being used nationally and internationally**
- **understand the perceived advantages and disadvantages of economic evaluations according to decision-makers**

Key terms

Reimbursement Payment by the government/health insurance company to the health provider, that covers the total or a proportion of the cost of the treatment.

Introduction

Economic evaluations provide valuable information about the trade-offs in the allocation of health care resources. However, they are rarely the sole basis for making decisions. Decision-making in the real world is much more complicated and includes considerations outside economic evaluations, such as fairness and justice, non-health benefits and costs, feasibility issues and others. The role of economic evaluation in policy-making is crucial because it supplements beliefs and expectations with research evidence of the magnitudes of costs and health outcomes.

In recent years economic evaluations have been growing in number and policy-makers in many countries have recognized their importance in the process of resource allocation in health care. In this chapter you will explore the process of producing economic evidence (the supply of economic evidence), followed by examples of evidence about the use of economic evaluations at international level, national level and local level (the demand for economic evidence).

Supply of economic evidence

In previous chapters you explored the methods of carrying out economic evaluations of health care interventions. In Chapter 16 you learnt about the guidelines that exist to improve the quality of economic evaluations and encourage comparability across studies. You also learnt that in some countries policy-makers require particular methodological approaches to be taken and, from working through this book, now have a basis of good practice against which to compare existing studies. However, when reviewing a range of economic evaluations you would find that variations in methodology and practice still occur (Hjelmgren *et al.* 2001).

A number of published reviews of the economic literature have reported on the quality of existing studies. Gerard *et al.* (1999) reviewed published cost-utility analyses and identified variation in the quality of reporting of comparators, in the clarity of effectiveness evidence, in the assignment of utility weights to health states and in reporting of sensitivity analyses. Stone *et al.* (2000) explored the costing methods of published CUAs and concluded that there had been no improvement of methods over time. Jacobs *et al.* (1998) observed a wide variation among studies in how they measured indirect costs. Walker and Fox-Rushby (2000) reviewed published economic evaluations of communicable disease interventions in low-income countries and concluded that appropriate analytic techniques had been inconsistently applied. However, more recently Neumann *et al.* (2005) reported that adherence to methodological and reporting practices in published CUAs was improving.

Is it reasonable to expect that the quality of economic evaluations would be associated with their utilization? Evidence on the impact of variations in methodology, practice and reporting of economic evaluations on their use and usefulness to policy-makers is discussed in this chapter.

Economic evaluations and health systems

Thousands of economic evaluations have been published. Although they can be time-, country-, setting and intervention-specific, it is possible to identify general situations where their findings can be used. Haan and Rutten (1987) identified two forms of use of economic evaluations that vary across different health care systems.

In systems where central control over planning and finance is possible, directives may be feasible so that economic evaluations can be used to inform, for example, the provision of specialist facilities like heart transplant services. Alternatively, incentives are more likely to be the preferred policy in countries with managed competition in health care. Such a model suggests that given the political will, economic evaluations may have an influence irrespective of the type of health care system.

Use of economic evidence at international level

The 1993 *World Development Report* and its companion volume (World Bank 1993; Jamison *et al.* 1993) suggested policies to improve health in low- and middle-income countries. These policies promoted use of epidemiological and economic analyses to establish a league table of health interventions ranked cardinally by health gain (in DALYs) per dollar spent. They also stimulated national and international debate on health sector investment as well as further research on the estimation of the disease burden and the cost-effectiveness of health care interventions. The second edition of *Disease Control Priorities in Developing Countries* (Disease Control Priorities Project 2005) will include updated information about the global disease burden brought about by tobacco, alcohol, psychiatric disorders and injury, in addition to broader health system issues.

At an international level, policy guidance on cost-effectiveness can only be a recommendation. However, when individual countries are assisted in sectoral prioritization exercises for World Bank lending projects, adherence to the advice may be greater. Bobadilla (1996) has provided one of the most detailed reviews of the scope of such exercises in low- and middle-income countries. In sub-Saharan Africa, available studies covered 8–40 interventions. In Latin America the broadest analysis (including over 100 diseases and interventions) was performed in Mexico in order to define a package of care for marginal states and areas with limited access to health services. Following an announcement from the Mexican president, this package of care was introduced.

In 2002, the *World Health Report* (WHO 2002) included findings of the WHO-CHOICE (CHOosing Interventions that are Cost Effective) project that were based on the generalized cost-effectiveness analysis. Whilst the extent to which policy recommendations were taken up is not yet clear, some of the proposed policies based on estimations of cost-effectiveness were:

- micronutrient supplementation (depending on the prevalence of micronutrient deficiencies, either vitamin A, iron, or zinc);
- disinfection of water at point of use in areas of high mortality to reduce the incidence of diarrhoeal diseases and treatment of diarrhoea and pneumonia;
- encouragement of safer injection practices (although care needs to be taken when extrapolating the effectiveness of behaviour change interventions from one setting to another);
- use of some types of antiretroviral therapy in conjunction with preventive activities rather than directly observed antiretroviral therapy combined with testing for resistance;
- population-wide salt- and cholesterol-lowering strategies.

Use of economic evidence at national level

In 1992, Australia was the first country to issue mandatory guidelines for health economic evaluations of pharmaceutical products as a requirement prior to reimbursement. Subsequently, there were similar guidelines produced in Canada, Finland, the Netherlands and Portugal. In 1999, NICE was established in the UK to provide guidance to the NHS in England and Wales on selected new and existing health technologies based on their clinical and cost-effectiveness. The Department of Health and the Welsh Assembly government are responsible for selecting the topics for the Institute's work programme. Decisions from technology appraisals conducted by NICE are mandatory for purchasers (but not necessarily backed up with additional funds), although clinicians are still free to follow their own beliefs about treatment for individual patients.

✎ **Activity 19.1**

The following extracts are an interchange between Richard Smith, the editor of the *British Medical Journal* at the time (Smith 2000) and Michael Rawlins, the chairman of NICE (Rawlins 2001). As you read them, prepare answers to the following questions:

1 What conflicts do you think NICE has to face when making recommendations?
2 What impact do you think NICE could and will have on patient care?

📖 **The failings of NICE**

NICE, which covers only England and Wales, began in 1999 with three main functions. Firstly, it appraises new technologies, including drugs, and decides which should be encouraged in the NHS and which should be held back. Its other functions are to produce or approve guidelines and to encourage quality improvement. The biggest push for NICE came from political disapproval of 'postcode prescribing': patients on opposite sides of the same street may receive or be denied treatment because they fall under different health authorities, each with different policies on which treatments they will fund.

NICE began with a blaze of publicity by deciding that zanamivir, a new drug for treating flu, would not be made available in the NHS. Its decision was based on the lack of evidence that the drug was effective in older people and others most at risk of serious harm from flu. It glossed over the fact that the same could be said for many, even most, treatments currently available on the NHS. Zanamivir's manufacturers, Glaxo Wellcome, were furious, and the chief executive threatened to take the company's research abroad. Last week, NICE reversed its decision on the drug, declaring that it would be available to at risk adults who present within 36 hours of developing symptoms when consultations for flu rise above 50 a week per 100 000 population. Just how easy it will be to implement such complex advice remains to be seen, but NICE boasted that the reversal of its guidance showed its commitment to evidence. A pooled analysis by the manufacturers showed that the drug would reduce symptoms in those at high risk from 6 to 5 days.

It's easier to say yes than no

When NICE approves treatments – such as taxanes for cancer – then there's little fuss, although many cardiologists think that it oversold the use of intravenous glycoprotein IIb/IIIa inhibitors in high risk patients who have had a heart attack, perhaps because it was overinfluenced by the drug companies' secret evidence. NICE's problems begin when it tries to deny treatments. It decided against beta interferon for multiple sclerosis and promptly found itself facing hostile publicity and an appeal from both the manufacturers and patients' groups. Its final decision will not be available until the new year.

One failing of NICE is that it's living a double lie. The first lie – which is as Orwellian as its name – is to deny that it's about rationing health care, which might be defined as 'denying effective interventions'. Denying ineffective interventions is not rationing; rather it's what the Americans call a 'no brainer'. The population is smart enough both to know that NICE is rationing health care and that rationing of health care is inevitable. The second, and related, lie is to give the impression that if the evidence supports a treatment then it's made available and if it doesn't it isn't. In other words, the whole messy problem of deciding which interventions to make available can be decided with some data and a computer. It's a technical problem. This lie corrupts the concept of evidence based medicine, which the BMJ has long championed. The evidence supports decision making, but the evidence can't make the decision. The values of the patient or the community must be part of the decision. Effective interventions have adverse effects. How can benefits be weighed against risks? How, for example, might an individual woman or society balance the probable cardiovascular benefits of hormone replacement therapy after the menopause against the increased risk of breast cancer? This is not a technical problem. Similarly treatments that are highly cost effective in those at high risk are also effective in those at low risk – but at a very high cost. Deciding where cost effectiveness ends is not a technical but an ethical judgement.

These failures with honesty may lead to the ultimate failure of NICE, which could be the inability to say no except in obvious cases. Beta interferon is effective in reducing the progression of multiple sclerosis in some patients, and donezepil is effective in slowing the progression of Alzheimer's disease in some patients. A body that is not about rationing and is concerned primarily with evidence might have to promote the wide use of both drugs within the NHS, whereas a body that was honestly about rationing might legitimately say no to both drugs. We shall see.

One off decisions unbalance system

Another failure with NICE is that it considers issues one at a time and is mostly concerned with what's new and expensive. A better system, like the one in Oregon, would look at all interventions. Otherwise a weak body that finds itself saying yes to most new technologies will encourage the traditional unjust rationing by delay (waiting lists), discrimination (against the elderly and mentally ill), dilution (two nurses on a geriatric ward at night when there should be four), and diversion (long term care moves to the social sector). Patients with Alzheimer's disease might receive donepezil but perhaps be worse off because they lose some of their nursing and social care.

Transparency is vital in an issue as difficult as rationing health care, and NICE has moved in the right direction by deciding to make its preliminary determinations public. Still, however, the process is far from transparent, and the suspicion is that political clout is as important as evidence in the final decision.

Probably NICE had to exist in order for us to begin to think about something better. A single body cannot 'solve' the problem of rationing, but Britain would benefit from a body that admits it is about rationing, works openly, uses evidence, looks right across health care, incorporates ethical thinking systematically into its judgements, is more distant from politicians and the pharmaceutical industry, and is directly accountable to the public. Let's call it CHOR – the Committee for Honest and Open Rationing.

Reply from chairman of NICE

Dr Smith has a continuing obsession (clearly shared by a few others) about notions of rationing. The use of the term has now become futile. It means such different things to different people that it would be better if it were avoided altogether. If he now wishes to define rationing as 'denying effective treatments' he is, of course, quite at liberty to do so; but his readers should be aware that the way NICE approaches appraisals is more sophisticated.

Second, readers should be aware that NICE takes six matters into account when considering whether to recommend the use of a particular technology to the NHS. These are:

- The clinical needs of patients in relation to other available technologies. This is obviously an overriding issue, and the evidence base for clinical effectiveness is crucial.
- The NHS's priorities. This is a relative, and not an absolute, criterion.
- The broad balance between benefits and costs. This incorporates both clinical and cost effectiveness.
- The potential impact on other NHS resources. This is particularly relevant where there are potential 'knock on' effects for other parts of the service.
- The encouragement of innovation.
- Guidance from ministers on the resources available.

NICE's Appraisal Committee, in deciding on its advice, is required to make a judgement based on its overall evaluation of these six criteria. In particular, issues around cost effectiveness inform, but are not the sole determinant, of its guidance. Moreover, before the Committee reaches its conclusions it seeks evidence from and consults with relevant professional and patient organisations. In the case of glycoprotein inhibitors, for example, evidence was sought from 'consultees' that included the Royal College of Physicians, the British Cardiac Society, and the British Heart Foundation. Furthermore, the Appraisal Committee's total membership now includes four individuals representing patient organisations.

I can also reassure conspiracy theorists that NICE has not received any 'guidance from ministers on resources available'. This criterion covers the possibility that, at some future date, a technology may meet the Institute's appraisal criteria but, nevertheless, be unaffordable in relation to the resources available for health care. It is not (nor should it be) the responsibility of NICE to decide resource allocation between health, education, transport etc. Those are political decisions that must ultimately be decided by parliament. Because the process the Institute follows is transparent, any advice it might receive on resources available would be apparent. Details of the process are published on the NICE web site.

Nor have we been given 'nods and winks' about the nature of the guidance we should offer. And even if we had, the Appraisal Committee's members are far too independent to allow themselves to be manipulated in such a manner.

NICE fully acknowledges it will, in the future, need to seek the views of the wider public where value judgements have to be made about aspects of its work. For example the Institute was asked, last week, to consider and update existing clinical guidelines produced by the Royal College of Obstetricians and Gynaecologists on infertility treatments. This may require us to consider not just the scientific and technical issues, but also value judgements about priorities. For this reason, the NHS Plan indicated that NICE will be setting up a Citizen's Council to address such difficult and contentious problems, and advise the Institute on some aspects of the guidance it might give. The composition and working methods of the Council have yet to be decided, but we accept that there are some features of the Institute's work that require wide public (as well as professional) debate.

Finally, the Institute did not recommend the use of zanamivir in 'at risk' patients merely because 'the drug would reduce symptoms . . . from 6 to 5 days'. We knew this, and made the evidence fully available, last year. Additional evidence (which is in the public domain) persuaded the Appraisal Committee that its use could prevent the development of secondary complications. It is disappointing that, despite the wide availability of information about NICE, Dr Smith recycled myths, misconceptions and inaccuracies without any apparent assessment of the evidence. Hence the need for 'evidence-based editorials'.

⟳ Feedback

1 There are a range of conflicts within the decision-making process including:

- balancing views of individual patient organizations and pharmaceutical industry with scientific evidence
- needing to provide timely decisions and yet review all material
- balancing concerns for efficiency with equity (postcode prescribing)
- being accountable to the public and wanting to use confidential commercial information
- providing guidance on individual drugs without having an idea of the overall budget (where is the incentive to reject?) or revealing a cost per QALY threshold value
- how is clinical benefit balanced against information on cost per QALY?
- balancing the views of politicians, the public and science
- internal and external views of the decision-making process – you may have other suggestions

2 It's difficult to judge the impact. Recommending an intervention may not influence practice if:

- it is not affordable
- there is not sufficient credence given to a decision
- the advice is complex to implement
- the advice did not account for non-pharmaceutical care (e.g. aspects of social care for the condition studied)
- a new intervention is not considered in terms of the opportunity cost of existing treatments (for which cost-effectiveness data may not be available) – in contrast, NICE may influence care if the converse happens or if patients become more informed and effective demanders of new technologies and if a new technology dominates existing options; you may have other suggestions

Use of economic evaluation at local level

There are now more than 30 years of experience in undertaking economic evaluations. About 70 studies had been conducted by 1987 (Drummond and Hutton 1987). By 1994 there were 147 studies and six years later more than 2000 critical abstracts of economic evaluations had been published worldwide.

There have been several surveys undertaken in the UK that shed some light on the use of economic evaluation by UK NHS decision-makers. Table 19.1 summarizes the methods and objectives of these surveys. A broad range of decision-makers has been approached in these surveys from prescribing advisers to directors of public health and managers. One of the common aims was to ascertain decision-makers' knowledge of economics as well as their views on the barriers to using, and actual use of, results from economic evaluations.

Table 19.1 Methods and objectives of the studies

Study	Sample	Methods	Specific study objectives
Drummond et al. (1997)	784 individuals (283 prescribing advisers, 400 directors of pharmacy, 101 directors of public health)	Postal questionnaire survey	• Ascertain decision-makers' knowledge of economics • Use of efficiency as a decision-making criterion • Sources of information on costs and outcomes used by decision-makers • Barriers to the use of economic evaluation • Actual use of economic evaluation results
Duthie et al. (1999)	17 pairs of NHS decision-makers (a mixture of managers and clinicians)	Interviews in pairs	• To determine the relevance and appeal of diverse health economic measures to different decision-makers
Crump et al.* (2000)	12 medical decision-makers in a health authority (4 medical directors of trusts, 8 locality GPs)	Individual interviews, focus groups	• Identify sources of information on costs and outcomes • Identify criteria used in making decisions about adopting a new treatment • Factors that would encourage more frequent use of economic evidence
Hoffmann et al. (2002)	12 decision-makers from 2 Health Authorities (managers and clinicians)	Questionnaires, focus groups	• Identify the sources of information on costs and outcomes used • Health areas where economic evidence can potentially be useful • Assess the role of the NHS Economic Evaluation Database as a decision-making tool and suggest improvements

* This study was part of the 'European Network on Methodology and Application of Economic Evaluation Techniques' (EUROMET) undertaken in nine European countries (Finland, Spain, Austria, Germany, Norway, Portugal, France, the Netherlands and the United Kingdom)

Activity 19.2

Imagine you are a decision-maker taking part in one of the surveys in Table 19.1.

1   What do you think the main limitations of using economic evaluations are likely to be?
2   Which characteristics of an economic evaluation would you consider to be the most important?

 Feedback

These answers will depend on your own experiences, on the decision-making structures and political environment in your country, and on availability of and access to evidence from economic evaluations. However, the main limitations are likely to focus on the quality and relevance to the decisions you make.

Table 19.2 summarizes the principal findings from the four surveys in the UK. There was some limited knowledge of economic evaluation among each group of decision-makers. However, confusion about and suspicion of key aspects of terminology raises questions about how well informed decision-makers are. Given some of the technical nature of economic evaluation, Drummond *et al.* (1997) found that only a third of their sample had some training in economics and knew that guidelines on cost-effectiveness existed. It is possible, of course, that the confusion about terms occurred in those without training and experience in economic evaluation.

Table 19.2 Study findings

Study	Knowledge of health economics	Actual use of economic evaluation results	Barriers to the use of economic evaluation
Drummond *et al.* (1997)	37% of respondents had training in health economics, 33% were aware of cost-effectiveness guidelines	Limited mainly to cost of drugs or potential savings to budgets	Concerns about validity of studies; multiple objectives pursued by decision-makers
Duthie *et al.* (1999)	'Mistrust of jargon'; ICERs, QALYs, WTP – not understood	(Implicitly) limited	Short-term contracting cycles and lack of transferability of budgets
Crump *et al.* (2000)	Limited	Limited	Inflexibilities of health budgets
Hoffmann *et al.* (2002)	Various	Limited, mainly cost-effectiveness of emerging technologies	Quality and generalizability of studies; lack of accounting for equity

The use of economic evaluation among decision-makers was not very extensive. The sources of data used were reported to be either studies undertaken by themselves or those identified in the literature. To assess the use of economic evaluations, respondents were asked whether they had seen particular published studies (11 real and two fictitious). Strong conclusions could not be reached but it was clear that the extent to which studies were known to decision-makers varied. Actual use most often concerned pharmaceuticals or emerging technologies and one important outcome considered was potential savings to budgets. The results from other countries in the EUROMET project supported findings from the UK; the cost consideration was accepted by all decision-makers and 75% felt that economic criteria should influence clinical practice to some extent. In the USA, studies of how managed care organizations and hospitals set formulary policies using cost-effectiveness analysis in determining policies show that awareness and use is increasing over time (Zellmer 1995).

The range of reasons acting as barriers to using economic evaluations is instructive. Whilst a key concern includes the quality of studies, others focus on the decision-making contexts. The main perceived limitation was that most published studies explored the cost-effectiveness of particular health technologies rather than health programmes. The limited generalizability of some economic evaluations was also a significant disadvantage. Other common reasons for avoiding the use of economic evidence related to the lack of expertise to assess the quality of cost-effectiveness studies coupled with doubts about their reliability. Some of this related to the sponsorship of studies, the assumptions used and the fact that savings were anticipated and not real. When faced with relatively inflexible budgets, short contracting cycles and the need to incorporate multiple objectives (such as equity), decision-makers can find that economic evaluations don't address their priorities or needs. Therefore, to encourage use not only is more explanation of the practical relevance of study results and more training in health economics required but there needs to be greater comparability across studies that are more accessible and that allow impacts on budgets to be estimated. It is also the case that assessment of studies by a trusted source would carry more weight. These findings have been replicated among groups of decision-makers acting under a wide range of conditions and different political and cultural systems in Europe and the United States (Zellmer 1995; Luce *et al.* 1996; Sloan *et al.* 1997; Crump *et al.* 2000).

Making better use of economic evaluations and making economic evaluations more useful

You have seen that so far decision-makers seem to have little experience with economic evaluations, one of the possible reasons being that researchers rarely address their questions. This is not very surprising given the relatively small number of studies in relation to the multitude of possible questions. Therefore, if published studies rarely provide a direct answer to the questions posed, what is their use? Some commentators on economic evaluation refer to its contribution as a 'systematic way of thinking' about problems or as a 'way of assessing proposals' for the use of resources (Drummond *et al.* 1997). Nevertheless, there is a need for further research to explore precisely how reading a published economic evaluation that fails to answer the specific question they had posed helps decision-makers.

There are at least two possible explanations why published evaluations do not often answer the questions posed by decision-makers. First, there could be a lag between a given topic being identified as being of interest and the relevant research being conducted and published. That is, the decision-makers are addressing the concerns of today, whereas the current literature addresses the concerns of one or two years ago. Certainly one might expect a lag between the publication of the relevant clinical research and the subsequent publication of the economic evaluation. Furthermore, another component of the lag could be the time span between the research being completed and eventual publication. Stoykova *et al.* (2003) explored the timeliness of delivering cost-effectiveness information about new drugs with established effectiveness and significant financial impact, in the context of NICE. Thirty health technologies assessed by NICE were analysed. Results showed that their effectiveness had been demonstrated in the preceding 12 years. However, cost-effectiveness evidence had been published for 21 (70%) of the technologies more than half of which were estimated using models. The good quality evidence on effectiveness lagged behind the first evidence by 1.4 years (95%, confidence interval 0.57–2.23), while the mean lag between the first evidence of effectiveness and the first cost-effectiveness publications was estimated as 3.20 years (95%, confidence interval 1.76–4.65).

The second reason why published economic evaluations do not often answer the questions posed by decision-makers is that the topics addressed in published studies are quite specific, whereas decision-makers' questions are often more general. For example, one of the main questions posed by decision-makers in Hoffmann *et al.* (2002) was 'How can we reduce the pressures on acute hospital beds?', whereas most of the evaluations located dealt with specific issues, such as hospital versus home care for particular medical conditions. Of course, these evaluations are relevant to the broader question but would require synthesis and extrapolation to move from the specific to the general.

Economic evaluation is largely driven by the availability of funding, which is much more plentiful for the study of specific health technologies such as new pharmaceuticals. Much economic evaluation builds on randomized trials, which tend to compare specific interventions rather than systems of organizing care. Also, it should be recognized that not every managerial or policy question is researchable, without further refinement and clarification.

Should a quality scoring system for economic evaluation be developed? In the study by Hoffmann *et al.* (2002), decision-makers appreciated better access to research studies and also felt that an overall quality score would be useful. Presumably the idea is that a published paper achieving a low score could be quickly disregarded. The first issue for health economists to address is whether such an approach would be desirable. The contrary view is that even a poor study, if appropriately critiqued, can be useful to a decision-maker considering a particular resource allocation problem. It is also somewhat ironic that decision-makers, who sometimes complain about the aggregation implicit in QALYs, are keen to have a summary score for the evaluation as a whole!

One of the issues raised by decision-makers was that many studies were undertaken in a setting quite different from their own or were quite old. In part, the seriousness of this concern relates to the earlier discussion about the use of studies.

Namely, if the study is being used to provide a direct answer to a question, it had better be relevant to the decision-makers' setting and up-to-date. On the other hand, if the study is being used to help structure the decision-makers' thinking about a given problem, direct relevance to the time and place may not be so important.

 Activity 19.3

Imagine you are a decision-maker in your country and you are experiencing pressure (from the pharmaceutical industry, patient groups or medical profession) to introduce a new widely advertised drug for breast cancer. Under the circumstances you have decided that evidence provided by a rapid literature review and an economic evaluation (within six to nine months) should be used to inform the decision. What approach to the economic evaluation would you expect applicants to recommend if you sent out a call for proposals to undertake the review?

 Feedback

The process should begin by clarifying the decision options. The approach would need to incorporate the results of a literature review into a series of economic models that compare the cost and effects of the new drug against comparators that are relevant to your setting (considering drugs of a similar class, usual practice, best practice and other surgical and nursing options). It would not be sufficient to simply list the findings from studies because the model would need to be specific to the proposed population group and subgroups of patients, reflect local resource use and prices, and would probably need to go beyond the length of time covered by existing data. The process may need to rely on experts' options in the absence of relevant data.

 Activity 19.4

In your view, how could the use of economic evaluations in your country be encouraged? Consider both the demand and the supply of such evidence.

 Feedback

Demand factors: decision-makers could be encouraged to acknowledge the importance of considering the economic consequences of their decisions, which would happen if regulators and purchasers were also involved; and if evidence were easily accessible and credible. Therefore external agencies might develop review criteria and a dissemination route that reduces the cost of acquiring knowledge (e.g. providing clear briefing papers and guidance) and reduces lag periods. A closer interaction between decision-makers and evaluators might increase the usefulness of evaluations for practice.

Supply factors: this will be determined by the availability of health economists and others with the relevant training and experience, and their expertise in the conduct of economic evaluation so that the quality requirements of decision-makers are met. Evaluators should also increase their consideration of the generalizability of findings in order to help a broader community of decision-makers.

Summary

You have learnt about the use of economic evaluation at international, national and local levels for setting policy and influencing practice. You have seen that the general lack of impact arises for a variety of reasons but most importantly because of a mismatch between the objectives of evaluations and the needs of decision-makers. Ways of increasing the influence of evaluations were explored.

References

Bobadilla J-L (1996) *Searching for essential health services in low- and middle-income countries, draft report for Human Development Department*, World Bank. Washington, DC: World Bank.

Crump B, Drummond MF, Alexander S and Devaney C (2000) Economic evaluation in the United Kingdom National Health Service, in J-M Schulenburg and VD Graf (eds) *The influence of economic evaluation studies on health care decision-making: a European survey.* Amsterdam: IOS Press.

Disease Control Priorities Project (2005) *Disease control priorities in developing countries,* www.fic.nih.gov/dcpp/about.html.

Drummond M and Hutton J (1987) Economic appraisal of health technology in the United Kingdom, in M Drummond (ed.) *Economic appraisal of health technology in the European Community.* Oxford: Oxford University Press.

Drummond M, Cooke J and Walley T (1997) Economic evaluation under managed competition: evidence from the UK. *Social Science and Medicine* 45(4):583–95.

Duthie T, Trueman P, Chancellor J and Diez L (1999) Research into the use of health economics in decision-making in the United Kingdom – phase II: is health economics for good or evil? *Health Policy* 46:143–57.

Gerard K, Smoker I and Seymour J (1999) Raising the quality of cost-utility analyses: lessons learnt and still to learn. *Health Policy* 46:217–38.

Haan GHMG and Rutten FFH (1987) Economic appraisal and planning decisions for health technologies, in MF Drummond (ed.) *Economic appraisal of health technology in the European Community.* Oxford: Oxford University Press.

Hjelmgren J, Berggren F and Andersson F (2001) Health economic guidelines – similarities, differences and some implications. *Value Health* 4(3):225–50.

Hoffmann C, Stoykova BA, Nixon J, Glanville JM, Misso K and Drummond MF (2002) Do health-care decision makers find economic evaluations useful? The findings of focus group research in UK health authorities. *Value Health* 5(2):71–8.

Jacobs P and Fassbender K (1998) The measurement of indirect costs in the health economics evaluation literature: a review. *International Journal of Technology Assessment in Health Care* 14:799–808.

Jamison DT, Mosley WH, Measham AR and Bobadilla JL (eds) (1993) *Disease control priorities in developing countries.* Oxford: The World Bank, Oxford University Press.

Luce BR, Lyles AC and Rentz AM (1996) The view from managed care pharmacy. *Health Affairs* 4:168–76.

Neumann PJ, Greenberg D, Olchanski NV, Stone PW and Rosen AB (2005) Growth and quality of the cost-utility literature, 1976–2001. *Value Health* 8:3–9.

Rawlins MD (2001) Reply from chairman of NICE. *British Medical Journal* 322:489, www.nice.org.uk/page.aspx?o=15423.

Sloan FA, Whetten-Goldstein K and Wilson A (1997) Hospital pharmacy decisions, cost-containment, and the use of cost-effectiveness analysis. *Social Science and Medicine* 45:525–33.

Smith R (2000) The failings of NICE. *British Medical Journal* 321:1363–4.

Stone PW, Chapman RH, Sandberg EA and Bell CM (2000) Measuring costs in cost-utility analyses: variations in the literature. *International Journal of Technology Assessment in Health Care* 16:111–24.

Stoykova B, Drummond M, Barbieri M and Kleijnen J (2003) The lag between effectiveness and cost-effectiveness evidence of new drugs: implications for decision-making in health care. *European Journal of Health Economics* 4(4):313–18.

Walker D and Fox-Rushby JA (2000) Economic evaluation of communicable disease interventions in developing countries: a critical review of the published literature. *Health Economics* 9(8):681–98.

World Bank (1993) *World development report.* Oxford: Oxford University Press for the World Bank.

World Health Organization. *World health report.* Geneva: WHO.

Zellmer W (1995) Comments of the American Society of Health-System Pharmacists. Presented at the US FDA Hearing 'Pharmaceutical marketing and information exchange in managed care environments,' 19 October, Silver Spring, MD.

20 | Critique of economic evaluation

Overview

Having reached this point you now know much about how economic evaluation of health care interventions should be conducted. You have been introduced to its scope and to many of its limitations. In this chapter you have the opportunity to stand back from the detail relating to methods and consider some of the criticisms, as well as the contributions, of economic evaluation for health care decision-making.

Learning objectives

After completing this chapter, you will be able to:

- **describe the main objections to economic evaluation**
- **explain the contribution economic evaluation can make to health care decision-making**

Criticism 1 – economic evaluation is unethical

Some people assert that economic evaluation of health care interventions is unethical. The information generated and its purpose implies denying some individuals treatments from which they have the capacity to benefit. However, if anything, a case can be made that not undertaking some form of economic evaluation is itself unethical.

It might appear that the problem of having to prioritize treatment and, by implication, not provide all care needed, is simply not having a large enough budget. But really it is more fundamental than this. Even if the primary concern of government or society as a whole was to improve health, it would not be sensible to go on spending on health care until there was no incremental health benefit from devoting further resources. However, there are many ways of improving people's health in addition to health care, for example, improved sanitation, improved housing, increased education and training, better nutrition, cleaner environment and improved transportation. The maximum improvement in health is obtained by spending in all these different areas so that, at the margin, they provide similar incremental health benefits. No economy will ever have enough resources to exhaust all the possibilities to produce a positive incremental health benefit. But even if an economy could exploit every opportunity to improve health it shouldn't because it is not just health that is valued.

Choices always have to be made about what care to provide and it is these choices that imply that some people will be denied treatment. Therefore it is ethical to let such decisions be informed by economic evaluation because economic evaluation recognizes that the opportunity cost of treating one patient is the benefits foregone by other patients.

Criticism 2 – economic evaluation is overly dependent on assumptions

A physicist, a chemist and an economist are stranded on an island with nothing to eat. A can of soup washes ashore. The physicist says, 'Let's smash the can open with a rock.' The chemist says, 'Let's build a fire and heat the can first.' The economist says, 'Let's assume that we have a can-opener . . .' (attributed to Paul Samuelson).

Economists are generally fairly willing to make assumptions. This is most evident in evaluations featuring economic modelling but it is also true, to some extent, of economic evaluations undertaken alongside randomized trials. Several concerns have been raised regarding economic modelling (Buxton *et al.* 1997) including the:

- inappropriate use of clinical data;
- biases in data from non-randomized sources;
- difficulties involved in extrapolation;
- very limited scope for validation of models; and
- opportunities for manipulation of the model to influence the results.

The greatest concern is possibly the last one. Analysts have considerable scope to exercise discretion with respect to the structure of the model and the values of the various parameters. This is primarily a consequence of the paucity and poor quality of the available research evidence but also of a number of unresolved methodological issues. The more complex that models are, the greater the scope for discretion. The resulting estimated cost-effectiveness will reflect the consequence of analysts' choices. Miners *et al.* (2005) found that ICERs estimated by manufacturers were significantly lower than those submitted by independent academic assessment groups.

Economists' response to a charge of over-reliance on assumptions is that their assumptions are generally based on the best available evidence. Even if the evidence is poor, decisions about whether to invest in specific health care interventions still have to be made. Good decisions can still be made with poor evidence and good decisions can result in bad outcomes because outcomes following decisions are uncertain. What is important, however, is that useful questions are set and the best evidence for helping answer them is used. Just because some information is precise and unbiased does not mean to say it is useful to decision-makers. It is far more important to ask the right questions rather than getting precise, unbiased answers to the wrong questions. Put another way – look for your keys where you lost them, not under the street lamp where the light is brightest.

Criticism 3 – economic evaluation misses too much

An argument can be made that economic evaluation is of very limited value because it fails to capture much of what is relevant to the decision it seeks to inform. The measures of health benefit, as you have seen in earlier chapters, are often fairly crude, and may fail to capture changes of importance to patients. Moreover, the emphasis on health outcomes will in some cases miss relevant changes in non-health outcomes.

ICERs – particularly cost per QALY – appear to be increasingly influential. They are deceptively simple. For example, the very strong distributional assumptions upon which they are usually based are easily overlooked. QALYs are summed giving each part of a QALY the same weight, that is, all QALYs are treated as having the same significance. No account is taken of any of the characteristics of those who are receiving the additional QALYs, or of whether the treatment generates a small gain for a large number of people or a large gain for a small number of people.

The argument that economic evaluation doesn't provide a sufficient basis upon which to undertake health care decision-making can readily be conceded. Economic evaluations certainly do not reflect everything of importance to decision-makers (Musgrove 1999). Cost-effectiveness might sometimes conflict with both horizontal equity (equal treatment for people in equal circumstances) and vertical equity (priority for people with worse problems) and decision-makers may want to take these criteria into account. In addition, they may want to account for managerial capacity and the size of the disease burden, if treating only part of a population is not politically feasible.

The argument for economic evaluation is not that it determines your choices but rather that it summarizes information relevant to such choices. It aims to let you make better decisions by informing you about trade-offs, such as between incremental health benefits and incremental costs. It has the potential for decision-making to be more explicit and transparent.

Criticism 4 – mismatch between what decision-makers want and what economic evaluation delivers

Some critics would argue that economic evaluation has not fulfilled its promise and that it has made a relatively small contribution to decision-making. This may be in part because they were not the right studies – the options compared may not be of interest or the costs and outcomes included were not relevant to the decision-makers. Alternatively, the results may not be available or sufficiently accessible when required. As methods of economic evaluation are not standardized it can also mean that results are often not comparable, which frustrates decision-makers. Finally, decision-makers can find economic evaluations are a bit of a 'black box' – they can see what goes in and the results that come out, but can't see how it works. Sometimes findings contradict their expectations and therefore they may ignore them – sometimes correctly (Brown 1999).

There are many barriers to the widespread use of the huge body of economic evaluations (Hauck et al. 2004) but generalizability is probably the key issue. How often do ICERs derived in one setting reflect the opportunity costs facing decision-makers in some other setting? There are many reasons why the estimates of cost-effectiveness may not be relevant and need to be adapted: differences in the population group for whom treatment is being considered; differences in the incidence of the disease; differences in the way the health services are organized and resourced; differences in unit costs; differences in clinical practice and so on. All of these factors could have a significant impact on cost-effectiveness. However, the paucity of research on how to adapt costs and effects appropriately is creating a gap between the knowledge available and the information desired by decision-makers.

There is a tension between researchers and the users of economic evaluations with respect to the methods of economic evaluation. The incentives for academic researchers are directed at refinement, development and increasing sophistication of methods rather than simplification, whereas the incentive for other researchers (such as pharmaceutical companies) is selling their products. Users of evaluations might prefer less sophisticated and ambitious models or models that involve head-to-head comparisons of competing products conducted in an unbiased way. Improvements in methods often do little to advance the cause of transparency.

There is also a tension in who is considered a user of economic evaluations. In some cases users could be considered producers, for example a pharmaceutical company may commission an evaluation from a consulting company or university research department. In other cases researchers may use results from another study to feed into a model comparing two interventions that have not been compared directly in a randomized trial. A third possibility is that a health care purchaser commissions a review with remodelling of results to answer specific questions to guide purchasing decisions.

The potential tensions need to be addressed if economic evaluations are to become more useful to decision-makers. Perhaps the increasing requirement to adhere to guidelines in the conduct of economic evaluation will go part way to solving some of the difficulties with comparability. However, given that each evaluation has a different purpose, Brown (1999) urges decision-makers to become involved in 'continuous and unreserved communication' about the design, structure and choice of outcomes within models in order to minimize the mismatch.

Of the four criticisms reviewed here, the last is the hardest to rebut. A more convincing case could be made for the value of economic evaluation if there was evidence of improved decision-making as a consequence of its use rather than just demonstrating that economic evidence *is* used. However, as with any contributing knowledge, it would be almost impossible to isolate unambiguously the contribution of economic evaluation to a particular decision.

Economic evaluation: success or failure?

Despite the concerns raised over the importance and relevance of economic evaluation, a strong case can be made that the application of the methods of economic evaluation to health care has been a considerable success. Over the last 20 to 30 years there has been a massive and sustained expansion of economic evaluation. The total number of studies was in excess of 30,500 by February 2005. In many countries there is now a requirement that the cost-effectiveness of health technologies, particularly pharmaceuticals, is considered when making decisions. Funders of clinical research and health services research are seeing a somewhat greater potential for, and relevance of, economic evaluation in proposals for new research. It appears that economic evaluation is being used increasingly to inform decision-making.

There has been a marked technical improvement in the quality of methods and conduct of economic evaluation. For example, there has been much greater acknowledgement that any estimate of cost-effectiveness is surrounded by considerable uncertainties regarding costs and health outcomes. As was emphasized in earlier chapters, there are uncertainties over the parameters of models and how the costs and consequences should be modelled. The handling of this uncertainty has been an area of notable advance. However, increasing sophistication of methods is not necessarily a reliable indicator of progress overall. The data analysed in economic evaluations has generally been increasing in both volume and relevance. For example, there have been improvements with respect to both the measurement of quality of life and increased availability of individual resource use data. However, it is still the case that routine data on longer-term consequences of treatment are rarely collected.

Economists are frequently to be found emphasizing not the numbers produced but rather the approach, the framework, the way of thinking. While there is some concern that the jargon is proliferating faster than the underlying concepts, it is quite clear that the economists' message has moved well beyond the discipline and influences the way people speak, and think, about health care.

 Activity 20.1

Write a 300-word editorial which describes the limitations of economic evaluation as a means of informing the allocation of resources in the health service.

 Feedback

You might want to make it appear unethical (remember not to mention opportunity cost). You will probably want to emphasize how little it tells you about the real concerns of decision-makers, its crude assumptions, and the scope for manipulating the results.

 Activity 20.2

Imagine that you have to make a presentation to a group of senior clinicians and health service managers. Your task is to persuade them that it would be worthwhile putting more energy and resources in to undertaking economic evaluations. What are the main points you would make?

 Feedback

You should emphasize opportunity cost and how economic evaluation makes the trade-offs explicit. Make it clear that the evaluation does not take the decision but is a means of organizing relevant information in a consistent manner.

Summary

You have seen how, despite the considerable progress economists have made in developing evaluation methods, there is still some way to go in the resulting evaluations having a major impact on health care decision-making. You have learnt about the four principal criticisms made by decision-makers and others and the response from economists. While there is still more to do to improve economic evaluation, considerable progress has been made over the past 30 years.

References

Brown R (1999) *How misused decision aids mislead policy makers*, working paper, Decision Analysis Society, http://fisher.osu.edu/~butler_267/DAPapers/.

Buxton MJ, Drummond MF, van Hout BA, Prince RL, Sheldon TA, Szucs T and Vray M (1997) Modelling in economic evaluation. an unavoidable fact of life. *Health Economics* 6:217–27.

Hauck K, Smith PC and Goddard M (2004) *The economics of priority setting for health care: a literature review*, health, nutrition and population discussion paper. Washington, DC: IBRD/The World Bank.

Miners AH, Garau M, Fidan D and Fischer AJ (2005) Comparing estimates of cost effectiveness submitted to the National Institute for Clinical excellence (NICE) by different organisations: retrospective study. *British Medical Journal* 330:82–5.

Musgrove P (1999) Public spending on health care: how are different criteria related? *Health Policy* 47(3):207–23.

Glossary

Allocative (Pareto, social) efficiency A situation in which it is not possible to improve the welfare of one person in an economy without making someone else worse off.

Average cost-effectiveness ratio The total cost divided by total effectiveness of a single intervention (where effectiveness is measured on a single scale).

Axiom of stationarity The assumption that preference for one intervention over another will be unchanged if both are either brought forward in time or postponed by the same amount.

Catastrophic risk The likelihood that there will be some event so devastating that all returns from a programme or intervention are eliminated, or at least radically and unpredictably altered.

Chance node The point in a decision tree where an outcome is subject to chance and to which a probability can be attached.

Clinical guidelines Advice based on the best available research evidence and clinical expertise.

Clinical or professional judgement The decision taken by a clinician as to whether or not a patient has a normative need.

Comparator An alternative against which a new intervention is compared.

Compensating variation The maximum a person is willing to pay (accept) to receive a benefit (loss) and keep at the same initial level of utility.

Compounding The process by which savings grow with the payment of interest.

Consumer surplus The difference between what a consumer pays for a good and the maximum they would be willing to pay for it.

Contingent valuation Survey approach to asking individuals to imagine markets exist and to give their willingness to pay (accept) for benefits (losses).

Cost-effectiveness acceptability curve A method of graphically displaying the results from a probabilistic sensitivity analysis.

Cost-effectiveness plane A figure with which incremental costs and incremental effects can be plotted relative to a comparator.

Cost-effectiveness threshold The level of cost per unit of outcome below which an intervention might be described as cost-effective.

Decision analysis This approach aims to identify all relevant choices for a specific decision and to quantify the relative expected benefits (or costs) of each option. The range of choices can be represented in a decision tree.

Decision node The point in a decision tree where a decision must be made between competing and mutually exclusive policy or treatment options.

Dimension/multidimensional One or many aspects (to health).

Diminishing marginal utility (of income or life years) Each additional monetary unit or each additional year of life gives a little less satisfaction than the last.

Disability adjusted life year (DALY) A measure to adjust life years lived for disease related disability, age and time preference.

Discount factor The present value expressed as a proportion of the undiscounted value.

Discount rate The rate at which future costs and outcomes are discounted to account for time preference.

Discrete choice experiment A quantitative market research tool used to model and predict consumers' purchase decisions.

Dominance When one intervention is both less costly and more effective than the comparators.

Effect size The average change in health scoring divided by either the standard deviation or baseline of change score.

Elasticity The percentage change in one variable relative to the percentage change in another.

Equity Fairness, defined in terms of equality of opportunity, provision, use or outcome.

Equivalent variation Willingness to pay (accept) rather than suffer a loss (lose a benefit) and yet be as well off after the change.

Evidence-based medicine Movement within medicine and related professions to base clinical practice on the most rigorous scientific basis, principally informed by the results of randomized controlled trials of effectiveness of interventions.

Extended dominance When one intervention is both less costly and more effective than a linear combination of two other interventions with which it is mutually exclusive.

Externalities Costs or benefits arising from an individual's production or consumption decision which indirectly affects the well-being of others.

External validity (generalisability) The extent to which the results of a study can be generalised to the population from which the sample was drawn.

Gold standard A method, procedure or measurement that is widely accepted as being the best available (nearest the truth).

Health-related quality of life How a person's health affects their ability to carry out functional activities and well-being according to their own subjective opinion.

Health index One number (usually between 0 and 1) that summarizes the relative value of several dimensions of health.

Health profile A graphical summary of each dimension of health measured.

Health state scenario A description of several (usually three to seven) dimensions of a hypothetical person's health.

Health technology assessment Systematic reviewing of existing evidence and providing an evaluation of the effectiveness, cost-effectiveness and impact, both on patient health and on the health care system, of medical technology and its use.

Human capital The characteristics of people that allow them to earn a wage.

Incremental cost-effectiveness ratio (ICER) The ratio of the difference in cost between two alternatives to the difference in effectiveness between the same two alternatives.

Intergenerational equity The fair treatment of future generations by preceding generations.

Internal validity (of a model) Accuracy and consistency of underpinning mathematical calculations with the specifications of the model.

International dollar The same purchasing power as the US dollar in the United States.

Managed care organization Health care provider that offers comprehensive health services based on explicit clinical guidelines.

Marginal cost The change in the total cost if one additional unit of output is produced.

Marginal productivity of labour The extra output produced by each additional unit of labour.

Marginal social benefit The extra benefit from consumption of a good as viewed by society as a whole.

Marginal social cost The cost that the production of another unit of output imposes on society.

Markov cycle The equal periods of time that the overall time horizon of a model is divided into and during which all information about people is held constant.

Markov state Markov models assume that at any stage in a Markov process a patient should always be in one of a finite number of defined health states.

Meta-analysis An overview of all the valid research evidence. If feasible, the quantitative results of different studies may be combined to obtain an overall result, referred to as a 'statistical meta-analysis'.

Modelling Simplifying reality and synthesizing data to capture the consequences of different decision options. This might involve simulating an event or a patient's or population's life experience mathematically.

Monte Carlo simulation A type of modelling that uses random numbers to capture the effects of uncertainty.

Morbidity This has two meanings: being ill and the illness rate of a population.

Mortality This has two meanings: being mortal and the death rate of a population.

Multi-way (multivariate) sensitivity analysis An exploration of the impact on the results of changing the value of two or more parameters at the same time.

Mutually exclusive interventions When implementation of a particular intervention excludes the possibility of implementing other interventions – for example, if one drug is used as first-line treatment for a particular condition this implies that any other drug cannot be used as first-line treatment.

Non-traded goods Services and commodities which cannot be traded on the international market. Therefore the cost or price is likely to vary across regions. Examples include utilities, buildings, domestic transport and some types of labour.

Observed/stated preferences What consumers reveal they want through actions or what they say they want.

One-way (univariate) sensitivity analysis An exploration of the impact on the results of changing the value of one parameter while keeping the values of all other parameters unchanged.

Operational (technical, productive) efficiency Using only the minimum necessary resources to finance, purchase and deliver a particular activity or set of activities (ie avoiding waste).

Opportunity (economic) cost The value of the next best alternative foregone as a result of the decision made.

Parameter An input to a model.

Parameter uncertainty The acknowledgement that a precise value of a parameter is not always known. This is also referred to as 'second order' uncertainty. It is represented in an analysis by specifying variables as distributions.

Pay-off Denotes the net value of the specific outcome represented by terminal node.

Pre-scored questionnaire A questionnaire that can help categorize the state of health dimensions and then use existing data to value the state.

Preferences This assumes a real or imagined choice between at least two options that can be ranked.

Present value The worth of a future benefit or cost in terms of their value now.

Probabilistic Any event is based on chance, randomness or probability – it can't be predicted exactly but the likelihood of the event occurring is known.

Probabilistic sensitivity analysis A method of analysis that explicitly incorporates parameter uncertainty. The defining point is that variables are specified as distributions rather than point estimates as in a deterministic analysis.

Psychometrics The science of psychological measurement.

Public good A good or service that can be consumed simultaneously by everyone and from which no one can be excluded.

Purchasing power parities Rates of currency conversion that equalize the purchasing power of different currencies.

Pure time preference An individual's preference for consumption now rather than later, with an unchanging level of consumption per capita over time.

Quality Adjusted Life Years (QALYs) A year of life adjusted for its quality or its value. A year in perfect health is considered equal to 1.0 QALY.

Reference case A set of assumptions and methods, which should wherever possible be followed by all economic evaluations so that different studies can be more readily compared.

Reference case A set of assumptions and methods which should wherever possible be followed by all economic evaluations so that different studies can be more readily compared.

Reimbursement Payment by the government/health insurance company to the health provider, that covers the total or a proportion of the cost of the treatment.

Reliability The extent to which an instrument produces consistent results.

Responsiveness The ability of a measure to detect a clinically meaningful change.

Scenario A brief description of a state of health.

Scenario analysis A form of multi-way sensitivity analysis, such as setting all parameters at their most favourable or unfavourable values in order to find how low or high the incremental cost-effectiveness ratio becomes.

Social welfare function This describes the preferences of an individual over social states. It is accepted to be a function of equity and efficiency.

Stochastic guess Pertaining to conjecture.

Study protocol A plan with complete details on the conduct of a study including tests, medications and procedures as well as study design.

Systematic review A review of the literature that uses an explicit approach to searching, selecting and combining the relevant studies.

Terminal node The end-point of a branch in a decision tree, where final outcomes for that path are defined.

Threshold analysis The value of a parameter is varied to find the level at which the results change (e.g. the level at which the cost per DALY reaches $50).

Traded goods Commodities that are available on the international market. In theory, all countries can purchase them at an international market price.

Transferability The extent to which the results of a study as it applies to a particular patient group or setting hold true for another population or context.

Transition matrix Summary of the transition probabilities between all Markov states in a model.

Transition probability The probability of moving from one Markov state to another at the end of a Markov cycle.

Uncertainty Where the true value of a parameter or the true structure of a process is unknown.

Utility values Numerical representation of the degree of satisfaction with health status, health outcome or health care.

Validity The extent to which an indicator measures what it intends to measure.

Value of information The monetary value attached to acquiring additional information.

Weighting (scoring, scale) A measure of relative value or the act of giving the relative value such as assigning a number or physical mark on a defined continuum.

Index